WHO Regional Publications, Eastern Mediterranean Series 32

Social determinants of health in countries in conflict

A perspective from the Eastern Mediterranean Region

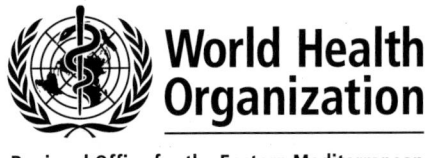

Regional Office for the Eastern Mediterranean

WHO Library Cataloguing in Publication Data

World Health Organization. Regional Office for the Eastern Mediterranean

    Social determinants of health in countries in conflict: a perspective from the Eastern Mediterranean / World Health Organization. Regional Office for the Eastern Mediterranean

p.- (WHO. Regional Publications, Eastern Mediterranean Series; 32)

    ISBN 978-92-9021-631-5

    ISSN 1020-041X

    1. Dissent and Disputes – mortality – epidemiology 2. Community Health Services - Mediterranean Region 3. Civil Disorders 4. Social Medicine 5. Disasters - Mediterranean Region 6. Health Policy - Mediterranean Region I. Title II. Regional Office for the Eastern Mediterranean III. Series

(NLM Classification: WA 295)

© World Health Organization 2008

All rights reserved.

The designations employed and the presentation of the material in this publication do not imply the expression of any opinion whatsoever on the part of the World Health Organization concerning the legal status of any country, territory, city or area or of its authorities, or concerning the delimitation of its frontiers or boundaries. Dotted lines on maps represent approximate border lines for which there may not yet be full agreement.

The mention of specific companies or of certain manufacturers' products does not imply that they are endorsed or recommended by the World Health Organization in preference to others of a similar nature that are not mentioned. Errors and omissions excepted, the names of proprietary products are distinguished by initial capital letters.

The World Health Organization does not warrant that the information contained in this publication is complete and correct and shall not be liable for any damages incurred as a result of its use.

Publications of the World Health Organization can be obtained from Distribution and Sales, World Health Organization, Regional Office for the Eastern Mediterranean, PO Box 7608, Nasr City, Cairo 11371, Egypt (tel: +202 2670 2535, fax: +202 2670 2492; email: DSA@emro.who.int). Requests for permission to reproduce WHO EMRO publications, in part or in whole, or to translate them – whether for sale or for noncommercial distribution – should be addressed to the Coordinator, Knowledge and Management and Sharing, at the above address; email HIT@emro.who.int).

Cover design by Ahmed Salah Mostafa

Printed by WHO Regional Office for the Eastern Mediterranean, Cairo

Contents

Foreword 5

Preface 7

Acknowledgements 9

1. Introduction 11

2. Approaches 14
   2.1 Definitions 14
   2.2 Sources of information 14
   2.3 Assessing the validity of the evidence 15

3. Profiles of suffering 17
   3.1 Who suffers and why 17
   3.2 Protecting civilians in conflict settings 18
   3.3 The regional impact of conflict 19
   3.4 Displaced populations: refugees and the internally displaced 20
   3.5 Border areas 21

4. The impact of conflict on health 22
   4.1 Mortality and morbidity directly due to conflict 22
   4.2 Morbidity and mortality associated with conflict 23

5. A social determinants approach to the health impact of conflict 26
   5.1 Major social determinants in conflict settings 26
   5.2 Other intermediate determinants 30
   5.3 Early childhood 30
   5.4 Health profile of children in conflict settings 31
   5.5 Older children in conflict settings 32
   5.6 Youth in conflict settings 33
   5.7 Social determinants affecting women's roles, capabilities and rights 33
   5.8 Displacement, loss of livelihood and community support 36
   5.9 Health systems that fail to support health 37

6. Views and voices from civil society 39
   6.1 Afghanistan 39
   6.2 Doctors for Iraq: a nongovernmental organization reporting from Iraq 41
   6.3 Resilience and social networks in the Lebanon crisis 43
   6.4 The Gaza Strip and the impact of the separation wall on life
       in the occupied Palestinian territory 44

    6.5 Surviving in Somalia 46
    6.6 Darfur 47

7. Addressing social determinants and protecting health
   in conflicts: everybody's business 49
       7.1 Strategies to protect health through a social determinants approach 49
       7.2 Interventions at the individual, family and community levels 50
       7.3 Cooperation to improve health care and access to care 52

8. Tackling the root causes of the problem 55

    References 59

In the Name of God, the Compassionate, the Merciful

Foreword

The Commission on Social Determinants of Health is a WHO initiative designed to address the social determinants that affect health outcomes and opportunities to enjoy good health. The Commission recognizes that action on these determinants lies beyond the usual remit of ministries of health, and that intersectoral action and collaboration between all concerned parties are needed to address them. Although the Commission established "knowledge networks", academic working groups to collate evidence on the links between health-related outcomes and social determinants, these topic areas did not include armed conflict. Yet, looking at the Eastern Mediterranean Region today, and in past decades, it is impossible to ignore the impact of these conflicts on health.

This review was written in response to concerns raised by Member States, by staff in WHO Regional Office for the Eastern Mediterranean, and by the regional civil society facilitator for the Commission, the Association for Health and Environmental Development (AHED), that conflict is a major social determinant of health in the Region and should be a direct concern for the Commission.

The role of civil society in the Commission represented a new kind of partnership for WHO, providing a global role for civil society voice, strengthening capacities among participating civil society organizations, and advancing the agenda of civil society in relation to the social determinants of health. From the civil society standpoint, the shared concern of AHED and their collaborating organizations for community-based action for health equity and primary health care, and a commitment to tackling the broader determinants of health, was expressed strongly through their concern for the plight of civilians caught up in conflict in the Region. As partners in this review, they were able to access local civil society organizations and knowledgeable individuals in the conflict-affected Member States who provided a grass-roots view of the daily fears and dangers of those living in conflict settings, and the impact these had on their health and well-being.

It is our hope that these responses and the examples of promising practices to ameliorate the impact of conflict will be of immediate value to countries and organizations concerned. In the long term, we also hope that this review will encourage those organizations and individuals who are able to influence the course of events in these countries to act in the best interests of their people and work towards lasting peace.

Hussein A. Gezairy MD FRCS
Regional Director for the Eastern Mediterranean

Preface

Six countries in the Eastern Mediterranean Region: Afghanistan, Iraq, Lebanon, occupied Palestinian territory, Somalia and Sudan, covering a population of approximately 100 million, are in a state of humanitarian crisis, demanding international intervention, as a result of armed conflict and/or occupation. A humanitarian crisis can be defined by four characteristics that have a profound adverse impact on health: dislocation of population; destruction of social networks and ecosystems, including destruction of livelihoods and health and social systems; insecurity; and abuse of human rights, including random acts of violence and destruction in order to spread terror, fear and uncertainty among a population. Many other countries in the Region are affected by the regional and global politics that fuel these conflicts. Thus, this publication also considers briefly refugee populations and border areas.

The objectives of this review are to: assess the impact of conflict on the health of people in affected countries of the Region; document how conflict affects social determinants, and thus results in adverse health outcomes; present the results of an innovative qualitative study that captures civilian suffering and resilience in a conflict setting, through collaboration with civil society organizations; identify some examples of activities and interventions that may help to mitigate the impact of these conflicts on the health and well-being of affected populations; and identify policy implications. The purpose of this publication is not to add to the documentation on the origins and perpetuation of these crises but rather to explore the impact of these crises on health status, and to understand the broad social and economic determinants and conditions that affect people's health in such crisis settings. How do the conditions in which the general population are living affect the health of that population, and which groups are the most vulnerable? What can be done to mitigate the adverse health impacts?

The social determinants of health in conflict settings reflect and further reinforce existing inequalities and the vulnerability of those who are disadvantaged because of poverty, marginalization and discrimination. The effect these conflicts have on health status can be explored to: identify the social determinants that are specific to the crisis setting; ascertain special dimensions of the more conventional social determinants that operate in such crisis settings; and suggest interventions that may help to mitigate their impact. The three social determinants that have been identified in this study which have a bearing on health and are peculiar to a conflict setting are: the loss of human rights, which can be seen as the first and most important social determinant in a conflict situation; breaches of medical neutrality, in violation of the Geneva Convention, Article 18; and progression from stress to distress and disease that results from constant, unremitting exposure to a life-threatening situation.

The WHO Regional Office for the Eastern Mediterranean, individual countries in the Region and civil society partners have expressed concerns that the particular social determinants of health associated with conflicts in the Region should be identified and explored. As a result of these concerns, the Commission on Social Determinants of Health requested a review from the Region. The Regional Office prepared the technical background by drawing on reports from civil society organizations in the countries and conducting an extensive review of published and grey literature. Where possible, sources published in peer-reviewed literature and official reports have been used. The authors have relied less on secondary sources found on web sites and in the printed media.

Conducting qualitative research was a challenge for all parties and required innovative approaches to draw up and implement a feasible plan of enquiry in a conflict setting. Many of the usual methods of qualitative research could not be rigorously adhered to because of problems of security and the need to protect researchers and their respondents. The reports from civil society organizations were submitted between April and May 2007 and the review covers events up until early June 2007, since when the health and security situation in many areas of conflict-affected countries has deteriorated even further.

In the face of immense challenges and in the absence of lack of adherence to standard guidelines to protect health, social determinants in conflict settings are the concern of citizens, local community-based organizations, international nongovernmental organizations, the media, academia and governments. It is hoped that this publication will add to constructive debate of the issues and to search for positive solutions.

Acknowledgements

This report was prepared by Susan Watts and Sameen Siddiqi, WHO Regional Office for the Eastern Mediterranean, in collaboration with the regional civil society facilitator organization for the Commission on Social Determinants of Health, the Association for Health and Environmental Development (AHED), in particular Alaa Shukrallah, Hani Serag and Kabir Karim. AHED collected reports from civil society representatives in all the countries covered in this review and the Regional Office acknowledges with thanks the Social and Health Development Program and Care of the Afghan Family research team, coordinated by Ahmaduddin Maarij; the nongovernmental organization Doctors for Iraq, project manager Salam Ismael; Aziza Khalidi, Higher Institute of Management, Islamic University of Lebanon; Jihad Mashal and Atef Shubita, Palestinian Medical Relief Society; the Somali Organisation for Community Development Activities; and Darfurians and recent visitors to Darfur who were interviewed by AHED.

The Regional Office would also like to thank the following people who, during the preparation of the paper for the Commission on Social Determinants of Health, read and commented on the draft: Jeannete Vega, Alec Irwin and Michael Thieren of WHO headquarters, and Sharon Friel, of University College, London, as well as Regional Office colleagues: Altaf Musani and Joanna Vogel. Thanks are also extended to Catherine Panter-Brick, Dawn Chatty and Olga Bornemsza for advice and encouragement.

Chapter 1
Introduction

Six countries in the WHO Eastern Mediterranean Region, covering a total population of approximately 100 million, are in a state of humanitarian crisis as a result of armed conflict and/or occupation. These countries are: Afghanistan, Iraq, Lebanon, the occupied Palestinian territory, Somalia and Sudan. Social inequality is widely recognized as an important cause of conflict, as well as unequal distribution of resources between groups, uneven economic development, and an unequal pattern of gain and loss prior to, and during, conflict. The social determinants of health in conflict settings reflect and further reinforce these inequalities and the vulnerability of those who are disadvantaged because of poverty, marginalization and discrimination [1]. However, recognition of the resilience, capabilities and skills of those caught up in conflict is a basis for positive actions to cope with extremely distressing situations and build a hopeful future.

Health systems in conflict settings are soon disrupted; prior to the conflict they may have already represented a financial barrier, and thus a social determinant hindering access to health care for a large proportion of the population. The health system is also often unable to ensure social protection for the population, and thus may contribute to pushing its users into poverty. The introduction of user charges at public and private health facilities has become standard practice in some countries, as has been seen in Afghanistan and southern Sudan.

The effect that conflicts have on health status can be explored to: identify the social determinants that are specific to the crisis setting; ascertain special dimensions of the more conventional social determinants that operate in such crisis settings; and suggest interventions that may help to mitigate their impact. The three social determinants that have been identified in this study which have a bearing on health and are peculiar to conflict settings are: the loss of human rights, which can be seen as the first and most important social determinant in a conflict situation; breaches of medical neutrality, in violation of the Geneva Convention, Article 18; and progression from stress to distress and disease that results from constant, unremitting exposure to a life-threatening situation.

The WHO Constitution, formulated in 1948, states that health is a fundamental human right and that living in conditions that result in poor health, and being deprived of health care are human rights issues. Maintaining human security is also a central concern for WHO, as noted by Kofi Annan, former United Nations (UN) Secretary-General in his farewell speech to the UN in December 2006, when he spoke about "the interconnectedness of the security of all people", "the global community's responsibility for everyone's welfare", "respect for the rule of law" and the "accountability of governments for their actions" [2]. An ethical and human rights viewpoint and the UN doctrine of the "responsibility to protect" also motivates the documentation of the ways in which conflicts, such as those in the Region, have a devastating impact on the daily life, health and well-being of civilians caught up in conflict [3].

In 1995, WHO established the Commission on Social Determinants of Health in recognition of the need to act to reverse the increasing differentials in health status, both within and between countries, which have been observed since the early 1990s. These differentials in health status can be attributed in large part to the differences in the conditions in which people live, and in their capabilities to lead healthy lives. Armed conflict results in life settings that produce high levels of mortality, disability and morbidity (physical as well as mental), directly or indirectly resulting from the conflict, when compared to health outcomes in otherwise comparable non-conflict settings.

The Commission recognizes the distinction between inequalities or disparities in health, and inequities. Inequities are defined as unfair or unjust differences in health status that are avoidable, and hence, can be remedied [4,5]. In a conflict setting, health inequalities are clearly inequities, in so far as differentials are the result of human action, rather than unavoidable biological or natural phenomena. A corollary of this distinction between inequalities and inequities in health is the recognition of WHO that health is a fundamental human right. This is currently expressed in terms of "the right to the highest attainable standard of health" [6,7].

The Commission on Social Determinants of Health identifies several ways of looking at social determinants. The structural determinants originate in the socioeconomic and political context at the country and global level. These affect power relationships that determine the distribution of power, prestige and resources globally and within a particular country or society, including those needed to maintain health and social well-being. These, in turn, result in intermediate determinants, the social relations, behaviours and psychological characteristics which can be seen as intermediaries between structural determinants and final health outcomes.

The structural determinants of health in conflict settings are especially important. They include the broad economic, cultural, historical, environmental and "political" determinants of health. All these determinants can be reflected in the intermediate, and strictly more "social" determinants, the conditions in which people live which affect their health status.

Thematic areas can be identified as starting points for policy action and intervention. These relate to specific life situations, especially groups or areas disadvantaged with regard to issues such as gender inequity, employment, urban settings, social exclusion and early childhood development, which are known, or suspected to be, associated with poor health outcomes and/or health inequities. The Commission's nine knowledge networks, based in academic institutions, were given the task of collating existing evidence for the impact of these thematic areas on health outcomes, and identifying the pathways through which they affect health outcomes. They were also mandated to present "best practices" and make some recommendations for tackling evidence for the impact of these thematic determinants on health outcomes [7].

The objectives of this publication are to: assess the impact of conflict on the health of people in affected countries of the Region; document how conflict affects social determinants, and thus results in adverse health outcomes; present the results of an innovative qualitative study that captures civilian suffering and resilience in a conflict setting, through collaboration with civil society organizations; identify some examples of activities and interventions that may help to mitigate the impact of these conflicts on the health and well-being of affected populations; and identify policy implications.

Chapter 2
Approaches

2.1 Definitions

This publication focuses on countries experiencing "armed conflict" and its aftermath; "armed conflict" is a better term than "war", as the legal definition of war is controversial. Armed conflict has been defined as "a contested incompatibility that concerns government and/or territory where the use of armed force between two parties, of which at least one is the government of a state, results in at least 25 battle-related deaths in one calendar year" [8].

In the Eastern Mediterranean Region, armed conflicts involve the use of armed force by the government of that country or an external state. They are fuelled by "collective violence" on the part of people who identify themselves as members of a group and by external political forces—governmental or nongovernmental [1].

Stated briefly, by the International Committee of the Red Cross (ICRC), "Territory is considered 'occupied' when it is actually placed under the authority of foreign armed forces, whether partially or entirely, without the consent of the domestic government. A situation of occupation confers both rights and obligations on an occupying power." [9].

At one time or another, all or parts of the six countries in the Region which currently or very recently have experienced armed conflict also experienced a "humanitarian crisis", an almost total breakdown of authority and security, which requires an international response to protect civilians, who are the main casualties.

2.2 Sources of information

This publication draws on reports from civil society in affected countries and an extensive review of published and grey literature. Huge quantities of grey literature and on-line resources of varying reliability currently exist. An attempt has been made to focus as much as possible on specific issues, such as the conditions of daily life and health for those caught up in conflict. Where possible, sources published in peer-reviewed literature and official reports have been used.

The collection of materials from civil society, using a qualitative research approach, was coordinated by the Association for Health and Environmental Development (AHED), a Cairo-based facilitator for civil societies in the Region. AHED staff identified nongovernmental organizations (from Afghanistan, Iraq, the occupied Palestinian territory and Somalia), and individuals (from Darfur and Lebanon) who were best able to provide information to give immediacy to the civilian experience of conflict that is often overlooked in body counts or in media reports [10]. Staff from the Regional Office and AHED compiled a checklist of major topics for key informant interviews and focus group discussions. The checklist included major health problems, access to health services and evidence for differential health outcomes according to gender, social group, age, occupation and place of residence. Questions on "coping strategies" reflected a concern for the skills, capabilities and resilience of ordinary people, rather than their vulnerabilities. The information was analysed in-country to allow for local interpretation of the responses. This avoided author bias by letting the country voices speak for themselves.

As a result of the short time-frame and acute problems of security, especially in Somalia and Sudan (Darfur), not all questions could be asked, and the original plan to hold focus group discussions could not be carried out in all countries. For example, the response from the Somali nongovernmental organization, the Somali Organisation for Community Development Activities, was sent in the middle of some of the fiercest fighting and shelling yet reported from the capital, Mogadishu.

2.3 Assessing the validity of the evidence

As conflicts, by their very nature, elicit heightened, often exaggerated responses and emotional reactions, it is especially important to evaluate evidence with great care. Accusations of partisanship are often used as arguments to refute disturbing findings about health and conditions of life in conflict settings. Conventional health indicators, presented on an annual basis for a whole country, do not reflect the impact of conflict on health status. Health indicators are required that assess the health impact of conflict over the short term, and in different parts of a country. They are often based on sample cluster surveys rather than reports from ministries of health. It is also important to move from body counts and disease indicators to look at suffering and human well-being [10].

Recognizing the often controversial findings of health and social surveys, and the special requirements and difficult conditions under which they are conducted in conflict settings [11], even those published in peer-reviewed journals have been critically reviewed. A case in point is the heated debate concerning a paper in *The Lancet* in October 2006, with its very high estimates of civilian mortality following the 2003 invasion of Iraq [12–16].

In the area of mental health, the definition of post-traumatic stress disorder is open to criticism for medicalizing a response to extremely stressful life situations, and thus rendering it subject to treatment with medicines [17,18,19]. Some observers, especially representatives of civil society, have stressed the importance of a psychosocial approach, but one looking at the societal responses, rather than those of the individual [20,21,22].

Civil society viewpoints are even more difficult to evaluate. They come from the grass-roots level, and are mediated by organizations and individuals sympathetic to these views. Thus, they often present alternative perspectives to those in mainstream media. The validity of these accounts is accepted as having been seriously and conscientiously collected and reviewed, under difficult conditions.

Ethical issues involved in collecting information in conflict must first and foremost consider the safety of researchers, those who respond to their enquiries, and other survivors. These issues pose a special challenge when documenting sexual violence, where police and military who are assigned to protect women could be the major perpetrators of sexual violence [23,24].

The authors have tried to face problems posed by the evidence by:

- declaring their interests, in terms of the rights of all people to health and respect regardless of religion, ethnicity and gender;
- acknowledging the right of people to speak for themselves, and to be listened to: hence, the concern for the views of civil society organizations;
- identifying all information sources when this does not put the lives of informants at risk;
- being especially rigorous in the assessment of validity and reliability.

Chapter 3
Profiles of suffering

3.1 Who suffers and why

A "humanitarian crisis", such as is experienced in crisis areas in the Region affects the most vulnerable populations and has a profound adverse impact on health: dislocation of population; destruction of social networks and ecosystems, including destruction of livelihoods and health and social systems; insecurity; abuse of human rights, including random acts of violence and destruction to spread terror, fear and uncertainty among a population [1].

In such crises civilian casualties are high and those who are fighting often have few scruples about attacking civilians. In such a setting, it is necessary to identify traumatic events that are likely to demand humanitarian action in the short term. It is also necessary to identify the resources and resilience of a population and how such capabilities can be harnessed for present and future well-being.

Conflicts develop within the context of longstanding inequalities and social conflicts, exacerbated by the breakdown of civil authority, and are associated with:

- competition for power and resources, such as land and livelihoods, food security (the ability to import food as well as to access local supplies), water and oil (the five countries with the largest oil reserves, and four of the top six with natural gas reserves, as of 2003, are in the Region) [25];
- cross-cutting local identities that reflect social, political, economic, religious, ethnic and cultural structures and divisions;
- predatory social domination, which occurs in especially vicious forms with the breakdown of civil authority [1,25].

Local identities that so often lie at the heart of conflict are fluid. At some times, and for some purposes, religious identity is paramount, at other times identities based on ethnicity, language, livelihood, or place of residence come to the fore. These identities are often manipulated by those in power. Sectarian labels are potentially dangerous, depending on who asks questions about identity and when [26,25]. Time series maps, such as those labelling areas as Shi'a or Sunni (as in Iraq), are often assembled by outsiders, and are usually contested and simplistic. They tend to heighten existing tensions and contribute to the political fragmentation of peoples who, in pre-conflict times, saw themselves primarily as "citizens" [27].

Other factors that threaten human security in the Region have been associated with the tensions of accelerating urbanization, and the large proportion of young people who need education, health care, jobs and opportunities for family formation [25].

Conflicts provide opportunities for intervention by foreign governments fighting wars by proxy as part of the "war on terror", or by actual occupation. They also provide opportunities for transnational companies involved in oil and armaments, and the recruitment of mercenary soldiers. Often, participants in the conflict accuse aid workers of political involvement. This challenges the principles of "operational neutrality and independence" that are supposed to protect humanitarian workers in a conflict setting. When security worsens, the departure of non-local representatives of nongovernmental organizations and multilateral organizations leaves local aid workers in an exposed position [28].

3.2 Protecting civilians in conflict settings

In the various forms of internal conflict experienced in countries of the Region, civilians are victims of forms of violence which violate basic human rights. Occupying powers have a legal obligation to respect the rights of civilians in occupied territories [9]. The 1949 Geneva Conventions apply to "war" and combatants and civilians caught up in war. More recent protocols are designed to "protect the victims of modern military conflicts". In such situations, it is unlikely that combatants would avoid injuring or killing civilians. Attacks on civilians are illegal if they are defined as "intentional", "indiscriminate" or "disproportionate". The Fourth Geneva Convention, Article 18, states that "Civilian hospitals organized to care for the wounded and sick, infirm and maternity cases, may in no circumstances be the object of attack, but shall at all times be respected and protected by the Parties to the conflict." [29] The acceptance by the UN of the "responsibility to protect" in cases of genocide, war crimes, ethnic cleansing and crimes against humanity was accepted at the 2005 World Summit and endorsed by the Security Council in April 2006 [3].

Human rights are grounded in ethical demands that exist without necessarily being supported by legislation, as stated by Amartya Sen, whose work on a theory of human rights has influenced the stance of the Commission on Social Determinants of Health [6]. Organizations such as Amnesty International, Human Rights Watch and Physicians for Human Rights document violations of civilian rights, and the serious and deliberate deprivations that can be defined as "war crimes" and "genocide". Afghanistan has an independent human rights commission which courageously reports on violations in that country [30]. Such evidence can be used as the basis for legal action or for humanitarian intervention.

Peace through health is viewed as a valuable initiative to explore ways that health interventions in conflict zones may contribute to peace. However, critics have regretted its failure to develop as a powerful force, as an approach that is strong on ideology but short on evidence [31]. Common themes in approaches to health as a bridge to peace and conflict transformation that are relevant to this review include: healing trauma; supporting adequate and equitable health care systems; and strengthening the social fabric of daily life that has been torn by displacement and identity conflicts [32].

The experience of health as a bridge to peace in the Region has included humanitarian ceasefires to achieve health-related goals which transcend the interests of all parties involved. These humanitarian ceasefires have allowed the administering of childhood vaccinations, especially for polio, as in Afghanistan and elsewhere; the delivery of medicines for children in Iraq; and the conducting of preventive measures for Guinea worm disease in southern Sudan [33].

3.3 The regional impact of conflict

In addition to the six countries in crisis in the Region, a number of other countries can be identified as being directly affected by these conflicts. The impact of these conflicts directly affects civilians beyond the conflict zones.

- Islamic Republic of Iran, Jordan, Syrian Arab Republic and Pakistan have been affected by the inflow of refugees from neighbouring countries;
- Afghanistan, Islamic Republic of Iran and Pakistan have open and insecure border areas with very poor resident populations, as well as refugees and insurgents.

Beyond the Region:

- the conflict in Sudan has affected neighbouring Chad, with refugees and armed combatants crossing the border from Darfur;
- the conflict in Somalia has drawn in Ethiopia.

3.4 Displaced populations: refugees and the internally displaced

Refugees should be distinguished from internally-displaced persons (IDPs), who remain in their country of origin, often in very insecure situations without any recourse to livelihoods or other rights. The Office of the United Nations High Commissioner for Refugees (UNHCR), following the 1951 Geneva Refugee Conventions, has been given the task of assuring refugees basic human rights in the host country, and preventing forced repatriation when conditions are not perceived of as secure; in the long term, they assist in repatriation to countries of origin [34]. Refugees fleeing conflict to neighbouring countries need emergency and long-term support. This places stress on existing institutions and social relationships in the destination country. In Iraq, by March 2007, UNHCR estimated that approximately 4 million people had been displaced: 1.9 million were displaced internally and 2 million had fled to nearby countries, primarily to the Syrian Arab Republic (1.2 million) and Jordan (750 000) [35]. Half a million of these refugees live in Amman and 1 million in Damascus [36]. The ICRC [37] estimated that 106 000 families were displaced inside Iraq between February and mid-April 2007. Table 1 shows the numbers of people displaced due to conflict in the Eastern Mediterranean Region between 2005 and 2007.

Palestinian refugees are descendants of those displaced as a result of the 1948 armed conflict between Israel and the Arab States. Within the occupied Palestinian territory, as of 31 December 2006, there were 1 016 964 registered refugees in the Gaza Strip, representing approximately two thirds of the 1.4 million people in the Gaza Strip, and 722 302 registered refugees in the West Bank, representing 28% of the West Bank population of 2 372 216 [38].

The large number of Afghan refugees in the border area of the Islamic Republic of Iran and Pakistan only has access to strained local health provisions, which often lack basic supplies, mental health services and maternal care for the local population. Until recently, nongovernmental organizations focused on disaster relief and emergency supplies for refugees, rather than on the long-term needs of the community and so few sustainable improvements in welfare could be made [39].

Table 1. Populations displaced due to conflict in the Eastern Mediterranean Region, 2005–2007

Country	Displaced population
Afghanistan (2005)	911 685 refugees [33]
Iraq (2007)	4 million: 1.9 million displaced internally and 2 million fled to nearby countries
Lebanon (summer 2006)	Approximately 1 million displaced of total population of 4 million; 735 000 IDPs and 260 000 fled the country
Occupied Palestinian territory (2005)	3 million refugees live in Jordan, 900 000 in the Syrian Arab Republic and Lebanon
Somalia (2005)	412 543, of whom 400 000 are internally displaced
Sudan (Darfur) (2005)	1 million: 841 946 IDPs and 317 462 refugees

Source: WHO Regional Office for the Eastern Mediterranean, Cairo, 2007.

3.5 Border areas

The long border area between Afghanistan, Pakistan and the Islamic Republic of Iran (where the international border runs through Baluchistan) has long been recognized as an unsettled area because of drug smuggling and the the unregulated movement of people. These conditions, together with the absence of cross-border disease surveillance, are not conducive to the welfare and health of those living in the border provinces [39].

Chapter 4
The impact of conflict on health

4.1 Mortality and morbidity directly due to conflict

In a conflict setting, the direct impact on health is due to death, injuries or disabilities caused by violence. The indirect impact is associated with conflict as a result of the complete disruption of daily social life and infrastructure. While such data are difficult to collect, those on mortality, and to a lesser extent morbidity, due to conflict are likely to be more accurate than those which are indirectly associated with conflict.

In Iraq, estimates of deaths during and after the 2003 invasion vary widely according to the source. The first epidemiological survey of excess mortality, conducted 17–18 months after the invasion, showed over half of the deaths recorded resulted from violent causes and more than 50% of deaths occurred in Falluja [40]. A follow-up cluster sample survey conducted between May and July 2006, identified an escalation in the mortality rate that surprised the researchers, an estimate of 654 965 excess deaths since the invasion, of which 600 000 were due to violence (the most common cause was identified as gunfire). The Iraq family health survey conducted by the Iraq Family Health Survey Group between January 2002 and June 2006 estimated the number of violent deaths as 151 000 (95% uncertainty range, 104 000 to 223 0000) from March 2003 to June 2006 [41].

In West and South Darfur, cluster sample surveys conducted by the staff of Epicenter, the Paris-based research division of Médecins Sans Frontières (MSF), identified high mortality rates. In West Darfur, in 2003: "in four sites surveyed high mortality and family separation amounted to a demographic catastrophe." The death rates (calculated, in the short term, as numbers per 10 000 per day) were highest among adult and adolescent males, especially during the destruction of settlements and during flight, but women and children were also targeted. During the period in "camps" the overall mortality rate fell but remained greater than the emergency benchmark (that is, double the normal mortality numbers for the Region, 1 per 10 000 per day) [42]. In South Darfur, in September 2004, in the three survey areas the overall death rate per 10 000 population per day was 3.2, 2.0 and 2.3, for each respective area, and mortality for children under 5 years of age was 5.9, 3.5 and 1, respectively [43].

Overall, civilian mortality in 2006 was the highest in Afghanistan since 2001, with at least 669 civilians killed in more than 350 armed attacks [44]. In the occupied Palestinian territory, 31 426 people were injured between 29 September 2000 (the beginning of the second *intifada*) and the end of May 2007, of whom 8112 were injured by live ammunition, 7101 by metal bullets and 6740 by gas [45].

Unexploded landmines and ordnance remain a serious hazard after the end of conflict, as people attempt to resume their economic activities. Cluster bombs break open in midair and disperse bomblets that explode on impact. During 2001 and 2002, Afghanistan had the largest number of reported landmine and unexploded ordnance casualties worldwide. Between March 2001 and June 2002, as in other affected areas, a high proportion of those injured were civilians (81%), most were males (92% were men and boys), and a high proportion (46%) were younger than 16. Overall risks were mostly associated with economic activities, children tending animals (and playing), and adults farming, travelling and involved in military activity. The small proportion of women injured probably reflects their more restricted mobility [46]. In Afghanistan, 25% of injuries due to anti-personnel mines during the early 1990s were among children under 16 years of age [47].

Cluster bombs were targeted at southern Lebanon by Israeli forces in the closing days of the July–August 2006 conflict, in defiance of international law against excessive incidental loss of life and injury to civilians. According to an Israeli media source, Israel fired at least 1.2 million cluster bomblets. By October 2006, more than 20 Lebanese civilian deaths and 150 injuries had resulted from the delayed explosion of these cluster bomblets, and rendered many of the fields and olive groves of southern Lebanon useless [48,49].

4.2 Morbidity and mortality associated with conflict

The morbidity and mortality that is indirectly associated with conflict is difficult to identify and to disentangle from those due to other underlying causes of poor health. This is especially the case in countries of the Region, such as Afghanistan, Somalia and Sudan, which have long records of poor health outcomes due to the combined impact of conflict, poverty and ineffective health systems. Environmental crises, such as droughts and floods in Somalia, and drought in Afghanistan, have exacerbated an already poor health situation. In all cases, precise data are difficult to come by because of prevailing insecurity and violence.

Rare longitudinal surveys are able to identify an increase in mortality over time. In Iraq, a cluster sample survey found infant and child mortality increased more than threefold between January 1991, when the first Gulf War began, and August 1991. The increased risk of death was found for all levels of maternal education and for all regions. The association between war and mortality was stronger in northern and southern Iraq than in the central areas and Baghdad [50].

In the Kohistan district, Afghanistan, a study in April 2001 identified a humanitarian crisis on the basis of their findings that the crude mortality and under-5 mortality rate per

10 000 per day was 2.6 and 5.9, respectively, representing, over a period of 4 months, 1525 excess deaths among the 57 600 people in the district. Most of the child deaths were due to diarrhoea, respiratory tract infections, measles and scurvy, reflecting underlying malnutrition. This study was conducted by Save the Children, USA [51].

Maternal mortality ratios in Afghanistan are among the highest in the world, due to a combination of persistent poverty and conflict, at approximately 1600 per 100 000 live births in 2002 [52]. According to a 2000–2002 reproductive age mortality study, figures ranged from 418 in Kabul to 6507 in Ragh district, Badakshan province, the highest maternal mortality ratio ever recorded. Even though Ragh district was not directly affected by conflict, it was affected by the general paucity of health services found in Afghanistan. It is in a remote region in the Hindu Kush mountains, up to 10 days' ride or walk from the nearest hospital with emergency obstetric care. Given the high total fertility rates, these figures translate into a total lifetime risk of maternal death of 1 in 42 in Kabul and 1 in 3 in Ragh district. On the basis of such figures, Afghanistan can be considered the worst place in the world to become pregnant [53,54,55].

Table 2 provides a summary of the major diseases reported to the Regional Office from conflict countries. Rates of HIV prevalence per 100 000 population (15 and over)

Table 2. Selected morbidity indicators for five conflict countries, 2006

Diseases notified	Annual number of reported cases				
	Afghanistan	Iraq	oPt	Somalia	Sudan
Cholera	144 605	44	–	97	–
Malaria	329 754	4	2	49 256	2 888 943
Poliomyelitis	31	0	0	35	0
Measles	1990	474	1	7	228
Pulmonary tuberculosis	12 468	2855	20	11 941	9986
Diphtheria	53	6	0	–	15
Tetanus	43	9	1	–	115
Neonatal tetanus	33	9	0	–	115
AIDS	6	2	1	–	418
Meningococcal meningitis	–	48	–	430	6487

Source: [52]
oPt: occupied Palestinian territory

in Somalia (870) and Sudan (1454) and overall prevalence of tuberculosis per 100 000 (286 and 400, respectively) are much higher than for any other country in the Region [56]. High rates for these and other communicable diseases reflect a breakdown in health services, including vaccination, as well as adverse living conditions that facilitate the spread of diseases.

Chapter 5
A social determinants approach to the health impact of conflict

5.1 Major social determinants in conflict settings

The two major structural determinants, reflecting the character of armed conflict in the twenty-first century, are the loss of human rights and breaches of medical neutrality. A major intermediate determinant is psychosocial distress resulting from the structural determinants, expressed in terms of a final health outcome—mental health problems. Thematic areas can be explored as guides to action and interventions (see Box 1).

The loss of human rights

The loss of human rights is the first and most important of the major social determinants in conflict settings. Human rights losses are also similar to those characteristics that identify a "humanitarian crisis" that requires international intervention (see Section 3.1). The right to live in dignity and security are enshrined in UN conventions and protocols. They are, as Amartya Sen reminds us, primarily ethical demands that make claims on individuals and organizations that are capable of taking action to guarantee such rights.

Box 1. Social determinants of health in conflict settings

Structural determinants include:
- the loss of human rights which are usually addressed during emergency responses but which also need to be addressed in the long term through building up capacities;
- breaches of medical neutrality which require national and international action and the involvement of nongovernmental organizations.

Intermediate determinants include:
- stress, distress and disease: tackling mental health problems in the social setting rather than through individual counselling.

Thematic areas as guides to action include:
- vulnerable groups: everyone is vulnerable;
- loss of livelihood;
- loss of community support and social networks;
- provision of, and access to, health services.

In conflict settings, the loss of these rights is most acutely expressed as:

- lack of security; a daily fear of the next assault on life and dignity; inability to protect one's family; vulnerability to bomb attack; rape; absence of water or food;
- displacement, movement from "home" place and the familiar; becoming a refugee or an IDP;
- loss of social networks and family structure that comprise the fabric and meaning of daily life and its social reciprocities; this also involves the loss of social roles that guide behaviour;
- loss of livelihood; and loss of daily activity, access to land and employment opportunities that provide for daily life and needs, resulting in extreme poverty;
- food insecurity due to loss of land and resources for livelihood;
- lack of shelter; a plastic sheet, the shade of a tree or a ruined home;
- lack of safe water and sanitation;
- lack of essential health and other social services, such as education for children;
- lack of communication, leading to isolation.

The lack of these rights results in a dependence on others and on aid handouts which produces a sense of helplessness and a lack of purpose in life. The daily assaults represent a withdrawal of rights essential for survival—security, shelter, food, water and health. They also involve a loss of the familiar, accustomed life and way of doing things which is profoundly disturbing, not only for the most vulnerable groups, but also for people who were accustomed to coping adequately in their familiar life setting. These rights were identified by Amartya Sen as "second-generation" rights that support human capacities to realize the kind of life that people would like to live. Expressed in these terms, as social, economic and cultural rights, they have been recognized more recently than human rights related to political expression, the right of free association, political participation and freedom of expression [6,57,58].

Breaches of medical neutrality

Breaches of medical neutrality comprise a second social determinant specific to a conflict setting. These are especially relevant for the right to health care, as combatants attempt to weaken the resistance of civilians by deliberately depriving them of access to care, especially at the times when they most need it. They are violations of the Fourth Geneva Convention, Article 18 [29]. In the Eastern Mediterranean Region, examples of such violations include:

- attacks on health facilities and staff;

- attacks on health care providers and patients;
- attacks on medical convoys and ambulances;
- barriers, checkpoints and barrier walls that obstruct access to care;
- the politicization of health services, resulting in discrimination in the provision of health care on the basis of social identity.

In Iraq, many other breaches of medical neutrality have been recorded. Armed men have entered hospitals, demanded treatment for their injured comrades or have randomly attacked health staff. Like teachers and university professors, health staff are captured for ransom, they are assumed to belong to families who can pay the ransom and are targeted also because they work for the government. Iraqi Red Crescent employees have also been attacked [37,59,60].

In the occupied Palestinian territory, the Red Crescent Society is the main provider of ambulance services. Between 29 September 2000 and 31 December 2005, they reported that 1905 ambulances were prevented from reaching hospitals, 36 drivers and medical personnel were killed and 457 injured, and 351 health facilities were attacked [61]. Furthermore, according to the civil society report, the blockade on goods entering occupied Palestinian territory seriously affects Palestinian health services, making it very difficult for the Ministry of Health to import raw materials for local manufacture or to procure medicines from outside the occupied Palestinian territory.

Stress, distress and disease

The progression from stress to distress to disease is seen as the third major determinant, an intermediate determinant that results from constant, unremitting exposure to life-threatening situations, the final outcome of which is a disabling mental health problem. Mental health in conflict settings deserves a prominent place in analysis as it is linked to extreme stress, especially as deriving from the structural determinant, the loss of human rights to security and basic needs. Poor mental health and the inability to cope with daily life are the cumulative result of deprivations found in all countries in conflict situations. As there is no universal response to conflict and its deprivations, there is no universal measurement of mental health [19].

In Iraq, in June 2005, after 12 years of economic sanctions and two wars, there were approximately 5 million people (20% of the population) experiencing "significant psychological symptoms" and at least 300 000 people suffering from "severe mental health-related conditions" [62]. Of the 2000 people interviewed in 18 provinces of Iraq in late 2006—a period of increasing insecurity for the civilian population—92% feared being killed in an explosion and 60% said that the level of violence had caused them to have panic attacks [63]. Such high levels of mental distress are likely to affect people for many years to come.

In Afghanistan, in 2002, a national survey supported by the Ministry of Health, the Centers for Disease Control (CDC) in Atlanta, USA, the United Nations Children's Fund (UNICEF) and other organizations found a high prevalence of symptoms of depression, anxiety and post-traumatic stress disorder, even compared to other populations in a conflict setting. Two thirds of the survey's participants had experienced multiple traumas, and 42% had experienced symptoms of post-traumatic stress disorder. People with physical disabilities suffered higher levels of anxiety (85%) than those without physical disabilities (69%).

The prevalence of mental health problems among females is usually higher than among males, and the same holds true for crisis settings. The national Afghanistan study also reported a significantly lower mental health status among women than among men [64,65].

Mental distress in children is common in conflict settings. In Iraq, in late 2006, it was estimated that over 90% of 1000 children studied had learning difficulties, mainly due to the climate of fear and insecurity [63]. In early 2006 almost half (47%) of 600 primary schoolchildren examined in Baghdad reported exposure to a major traumatic event in the previous two years, with 17% of girls and 9% of boys having symptoms of post-traumatic stress disorder [66]. In occupied Palestinian territory, between 2002 and 2003, among boys and girls between 6 and 16 years of age, girls were more affected than boys, with 58% identified as suffering from severe post-traumatic stress disorder. Symptoms were related to both the extent of exposure to violence and the family setting, showing that military violence affected the ability of the family and home to protect children [67,68,69,70]. In light of the debate about post-traumatic stress disorder and the danger of medicalizing conditions that arise in extremely stressful situations (see Section 2.3), Giacaman et al explore the collective, as well as the individual impact of trauma on youth, and the survival of values that are central to the quality of life [71,72].

As each society is likely to interpret their experiences differently, and have different ways of expressing them, a more nuanced, and less biomedical approach to psychosocial distress may yield useful insights that reflect what those involved feel and how they express themselves. In Darfur, researchers from a nongovernmental organization, the Tear Fund, found that most of those interviewed interpreted their experiences of distress in terms of the social body, rather than the "self". For them what counted was the effect on the social life of their community of fleeing from their villages, and the loss of dignity and of the social roles they had enjoyed in their villages [20]. Social support, essential for mental well-being, is provided in a stable community setting. When this collapses, individuals suffer severe mental stress. For example, Iraqi asylum seekers were more likely to suffer from depression due to a lack of social support, than from having been subject to torture. "Perhaps the primary impact of war on victims is through their witnessing the destruction of a social world embodying their history, identity and living values" [19].

5.2 Other intermediate determinants

Guidance for actions and interventions to improve health outcomes requires an analysis of the health and social status of groups usually regarded as vulnerable, such as children, women or older people. But in conflict settings everyone, in one way or another, is vulnerable. Depending on the setting, members of these groups are vulnerable to violence as actual or perceived combatants or as bystanders; to malnutrition; to lack of social capital; to loss of livelihoods and meaningful activities; and to lack of access to health care.

5.3 Early childhood

In emergency settings, children under 5 years of age are most vulnerable, very often living and dying without adequate nutrition and health care in unhygienic environments. The commonest causes of death and illness are the same as those usually experienced in low-income countries: diarrhoeal diseases, respiratory infections, measles and malnutrition. Children and young people often comprise the highest proportion of the population in refugee and IDP camps, and are exposed to risks over which they have little control [47,73].

The social determinants affecting children in crisis settings are the same as those affecting children in low-income countries: (1) lack of safe water and sanitation; poor quality housing; (2) poor nutrition; and (3) lack of access to health services. In conflict settings, these social determinants influence the health, opportunities for social and intellectual development and quality of life of children even more, as they operate in an environment in which the basic rights of children have deteriorated due to:

- lack of security and family support, so essential during the first 5 years in providing a stable foundation for the rest of life;
- immediate threats to security during occupation, fighting, etc.; experience of traumatic events;
- lack of opportunity to learn social skills through social interaction with family and peers;
- lack of opportunity to play as a way of developing social and motor skills.

Conflict may result in the breakdown of the family unit, which has a negative impact on the development of children. As the social fabric of society breaks down, especially at the level of the family, children are denied lasting relationships with parents and other carers, siblings and other kin, which impedes their normal development, in terms of forming social relationships based on trust. Children taken in by extended family members or who have even one immediate family member are less likely to experience the extreme negative effects of family breakdown. Children who lose their families and other social links are more vulnerable to recruitment for military activities [74,75].

5.4 Health profile of children in conflict settings

In conflict settings, therefore, young children become vulnerable to major health risks usually associated with poverty, namely malnutrition and infectious diseases. Causes of mortality and morbidity often provide indications of the particular risks for children in crisis settings. For example, the survey in Kohistan district, Afghanistan, in April 2001, revealed a high mortality rate among children under 5 years of age. Most deaths were from:

- diarrhoea (25%): reflecting a lack of access to safe water;
- respiratory tract infections (19.4%): reflecting a lack of access to health facilities and appropriate medicines;
- measles (15.7%): pointing to failure of the Expanded Programme on Immunization (EPI);
- scurvy (6.5%): pointing to malnutrition [51].

Malnutrition in children under 5 years of age is a good indicator of changing health status among a vulnerable group, and is relatively easy to identify. Indicators of stunting, underweight and wasting are often available in national surveys, such as demographic and health surveys or multiple indicator cluster surveys. Long-term chronic malnutrition, or stunting, is often highlighted as it is likely to result in long-term health damage.

In Iraq, three nutrition surveys conducted between 1996 and 1997, which covered all of Iraq, found alarming rates of malnutrition among children after implementation of the UN Oil-for-Food programme in December 1996. Almost one third (32%) of children under 5 years of age were stunted or chronically malnourished, an increase of 72% since pre-war 1991 surveys, and almost one quarter (23.4%) were underweight. Some regions suffered more severely than others; the 1997 Multiple Indicator Cluster Survey found that almost half of children under 5 years of age in the governorate of Missan, in eastern Iraq, were malnourished [76]. Multiple Indicator Cluster Surveys for 2000 and 2006 showed continued chronic malnutrition (stunting), 22% and 21.4% for each year, respectively [77,78]. A survey conducted in Baghdad just after the war in 2003 found 16% of children were stunted [79]. Even higher rates of stunting (63.7% of children aged between 6 and 59 months) were found in Kohistan, Afghanistan, in 2002, after three years of civil war and drought [51].

Where children suffer severe acute malnutrition (a weight-for-height of three standard deviation scores (SDs) or more below the mean reference value), pilot studies have demonstrated the value of providing locally ready-to-use high-energy foods that minimize the need for hospital care, so scarce in conflict settings. This strategy has now been formally adopted by WHO and UNICEF for all community-based settings in which children suffer from severe acute malnutrition [80,81,82]. Infectious diseases, such as diarrhoeal diseases, acute respiratory infections, and, to a lesser extent, vaccine-preventable diseases, become major causes of morbidity (and mortality) among children in conflict settings, especially among refugees and IDPs. One camp in Darfur recorded a 50% weekly attack rate of diarrhoea among children [43]. As noted above, two thirds of infant deaths in one district of Afghanistan were caused by infectious diseases; in Afghanistan such tragedies are the result of long-term poverty, compounded by conflict which destroys the ability of the country to deliver effective health care [51].

In contrast, in occupied Palestinian territory, as of June 2006 (before the July–August conflict), only 6.6% of infant mortality was caused by infectious diseases. Other health status indicators also appeared to have held up well. As of mid-2006, the immunization programme was functioning well, with coverage of more than 95% for diphtheria, pertussis and tetanus (DPT), hepatitis B and measles, mumps and rubella (MMR) [83].

In the occupied Palestinian territory, in spite of the long-term chronic crisis, child health trends have improved. This has been attributed to the ability of the health system to deliver care under difficulties and the high level of motivation of the national staff, thus contributing to the control of major childhood infectious diseases, the maintenance of immunization and oral rehydration programmes, and an increase in the number of deliveries taking place in hospitals. The high educational status of the population has also been identified as supporting child health. Whether or not these health indicators can hold up in the long run is a moot point, given recent assaults on health services and deteriorating security. Recent evidence indicates that chronic malnutrition among children has been increasing, suggesting that food security problems are affecting children's health [83].

5.5 Older children in conflict settings

In emergency settings, children may adopt new roles; no longer in school, they may be helping to provide food and care for the family or for younger siblings and young girls may be mothers. Some boys as young as 12 years of age may be abducted or "voluntarily" join rebel groups and be given arms, and girls have been forced into various forms of sexual slavery, as reported since early 2004 in Darfur [84]. UNICEF is now working to reintegrate former child soldiers in southern Sudan into society, and provide them with education, employment skills and counselling. The resilience of these children was noted to be remarkable [85]. Yet, it appears that the resilience and strengths of children are rarely acknowledged in conflict settings, as they undertake what are often seen as adult roles or are engaged in the fighting. Human rights are not confined to adults; children too, have the right to be listened to, and to participate in health decisions that affect them [73]. At the same time, it is important to appreciate the wider context within which children might be directly involved in conflict and move beyond the condemnation of local combatants who allow these conditions to exist. This involves understanding the ways in which external forces, such as the growth in arms sales, the development of new kinds of small arms, and the impoverishment of whole countries affect the local setting in which children become combatants [86].

5.6 Youth in conflict settings

Youth comprise a larger proportion of the population in the Region than in many other parts of the world. Whether completing, or failing to complete, their schooling, they are faced with high levels of unemployment, which also affects their prospects of marriage. In the Region "youth" often includes all those under the age of 30. Almost three quarters of the population of the occupied Palestinian territory (72.3%) are under the age of 30. This age group is vastly over-represented in conflict casualties. Between the beginning of the second *intifada* on 29 September 2000 and 31 May 2007, 2644 males between the ages of 18 and 29 and 45 females resident in the occupied Palestinian territory were killed by enemy fire; this 10-year cohort represented 56% of 4504 deaths due to enemy fire [87]. Palestinian children and adolescents are active and politically aware, and there is a need to understand the forces that drive political street activism and to provide opportunities for alternative activities [88].

5.7 Social determinants affecting women's roles, capabilities and rights

Conflict and its attendant trauma often require that women undertake new social and economic roles. These roles may strengthen women if they are able to take advantage of opportunities to provide for their families. Alternatively, they may become more vulnerable, if they are isolated and exposed to violence and lack of resources. Women and children comprise a high proportion of displaced people; about two thirds of displaced people in Iraq are women and children, often in female-headed households [38].

New roles for women may strengthen their ability to cope in stressful situations, especially if they are able to act independently when they are separated from their husbands or from male relatives. Ways in which women creatively respond to crises include: maintaining social capital and social networks in crisis; working together for mutual support; and establishing and joining civil society organizations to protect themselves and their rights.

For social and physiological reasons, exposure to violence and reactions to it differ between men and women. Women are more commonly exposed to sexual and domestic violence, while men are exposed to direct military and civilian violence. Often women suffer from different symptoms and from more severe mental distress as a result of personally experiencing or seeing violence than men do. A study in the Gaza Strip found the lifetime occurrence of at least one traumatic event was higher among men (86%) than among women (44%), yet women showed higher levels of psychiatric distress, especially anxiety disorder (but not post-traumatic stress disorder). These are similar to findings of exposure to violence in non-conflict settings [89]. Another study in the occupied Palestinian territory found that women have higher rates of depression, even with lower exposure to violence, while boys and men tend to exhibit aggressive behaviour and use abusive language [21].

The loss of security, as a human right, is felt especially by women, who become vulnerable to rape which is used as a weapon of war. Women are seen by the military and insurgents as part and parcel of the land that must be subdued, a reward and encouragement, and a means of undermining the morale of men who can no longer protect them. Rape is also a deprivation of women's most precious right—control over their own bodies—as well as a violation of the whole social order. Social stigma associated with rape means that many women are unwilling to report an assault: children of rape are often unacknowledged by kin and the mother may be ostracized [90,91]. Reliable reports of assault in Darfur include: violence when women leave camps to collect firewood to sell or use for cooking [24] and sexual assaults leading to physical injuries [92].

Intrafamily violence is a long-standing problem in many countries. It is exacerbated in conflict situations, as in the occupied Palestinian territory, when people's tempers are daily on edge. Laws in force in the West Bank and the Gaza Strip, and in other areas of the Region, do not protect women and girls from domestic violence, indeed they often condone practices such as honour killing [93].

New social roles may be forced on women in a conflict setting or valued roles may be lost. For example, many Afghani women suffered under the Taliban regime which severely limited women's authority and independence. Women were not allowed to work outside the home and girls were banned from school. Gender boundaries became stronger among strangers, adversely affecting the status of migrants and those in refugee camps [94]. Researchers from Physicians for Human Rights found that policies were detrimental to the health, needs and interests of Afghani women. The majority of respondents reported a decline in physical and mental health status and access to health care. Many reported that family members were killed (84%) or detained and abused (69%), and many reported extreme restrictions on social activities [95, 96]. A national study conducted by the CDC in late 2002, after the new government took office, found high levels of mental ill-health among women [64, 65].

The social determinants of maternal mortality are indirectly associated with conflict; a worsening of the existing circumstances, such as long-standing poverty and limitations on women's mobility. Countries, such as Afghanistan and Somalia, have recorded some of the highest maternal mortality ratios, an estimate of 1600 per 100 000 live births for both countries [52]. The authors of a study, affiliated with Physicians for Human Rights, based in Boston, USA, identified the specific social determinants involved in high maternal mortality in Afghanistan (see Box 2). They interpreted such high maternal mortality ratios as a deprivation of women's human rights, rights to health care, education and the freedom to make decisions for themselves [97 see also 53,55].

Adult males are usually recognized as vulnerable in their role as combatants. However, in recent conflicts civilian adult males are also vulnerable. In occupied Palestinian territory men must travel to, and seek, work. They endure many stressful and dangerous encounters at checkpoints. In Iraq, Doctors for Iraq reported that men were the main casualties in the conflict, with civilian males directly affected by violence, especially kidnapping and assassination.

Women and men aged 60 and older living in war-affected areas in Lebanon (during the July–August 2006 conflict) experienced psychosomatic symptoms: 47.7% of men and 48% of women complained of exhaustion; insomnia and depression were next on the list. These problems added to the normal challenges of physical ageing and chronic disease [98].

Prisoners are vulnerable to deteriorating prison conditions, as noted by the nongovernmental organization, Doctors for Iraq. IDPs are often more vulnerable than refugees even when in camps, as they may be more exposed to violence and experience more difficulties in providing for daily life than refugees. People with physical disabilities are vulnerable as health systems in many affected countries lack the ability to deal with their problems; they face a transformed life in conditions of social exclusion. The vulnerability of street children, orphans, beggars and the unemployed is noted in civil society reports.

Box 2. Social determinants of maternal mortality in Afghanistan

In 2002, after 20 years of war, a survey in Herat province found the determinants of high maternal mortality to include:

- rural residence: 92% of maternal deaths occurred in rural areas;
- age at marriage: mean age at marriage (15 years);
- lack of education: 94% of respondents had less than 1 year of formal education;
- barriers for women in obtaining permission to seek health care;
- lack of primary care and low utilization of available health care:
  - only 11% of women reported receiving prenatal care;
  - less than 1% of women reported that a trained health care worker attended their delivery.
- lack of availability of hospital care: only 17 of the 27 listed health facilities were functional and only five provided essential obstetric care [53].

5.8 Displacement, loss of livelihood and community support

Many people living in areas of conflict have lost their livelihoods due to a combination of: forced population movement (in Darfur, Iraq, the occupied Palestinian territory); deliberate destruction of farmland and homes (in Darfur, Lebanon, the occupied Palestinian territory); barriers denying access to jobs (Palestinians working in Israel or on the wrong side of the separation wall); and fear and flight when livelihoods are threatened (government workers in Afghanistan and Iraq).

Livelihoods have been affected in Afghanistan and southern Lebanon by the widespread presence of unexploded ordnance which civil society reports noted makes it dangerous for anyone to move away from well-trodden paths, hence, to visit their farms and orchards, or tend their animals.

According to the Palestinian civil society report Palestinians have experienced a gradual erosion of their rights to livelihood due to the extension of checkpoints, barriers and the separation wall, which have prevented people from going to their fields or their work sites in nearby areas of the occupied Palestinian territory or in Israel. Farmers have been unable to take their produce to the markets, or have been forced to watch it rot as their trucks wait to pass through a checkpoint.

As of January 2007 in the occupied Palestinian territory, approximately 70% of the workforce in the Gaza Strip were either out of work or were working without pay (due to non-payment of salaries of public sector employees, especially in the health and education sectors). More than 70% of the population was living below the poverty line [99]. The crisis in early 2006 prompted the Food and Agriculture Organization of the United Nations (FAO) and the World Food Programme (WFP) to conduct a food security analysis in the West Bank and the Gaza Strip. The study found that one third of the population was food insecure and one third food secure, with the rest hovering in between. These findings were similar to those of the 2003 food security assessment, which found approximately 4 out of 10 people were food insecure, with 30% under threat of becoming food insecure. One reason for the situation not becoming so much worse between the time that the two surveys were conducted was continuing family support and the resilience of the population, which was further stretched during and after the summer 2006 conflict. Food insecurity in 2006 was markedly higher among refugees who lived in camps (44.7%). As almost half (46%) of the Palestinian population are children under 14 years of age, the impact of food insecurity is proportionally more severe [100, 101].

5.9 Health systems that fail to support health

Health systems in conflict settings are among the first to become disrupted in what are now increasingly being called 'fragile states'. Often health systems in such countries were already weak prior to the conflict and subsequently became dysfunctional as a result of it. Under such circumstances health systems become a financial barrier, and thus a social determinant hindering access to health care for a large proportion of the affected population. In addition to its inability to protect health, the health system is also unable to ensure the social protection of the population, and thus may contribute to pushing its users into poverty.

In many cases health services may exist on paper but have ceased to provide health services to the people in their catchment area. For example, in Afghanistan, as hospitals and community mental health centres have ceased to function, people suffering from mental illness have largely been unable to access care, and emergency obstetric care is largely absent [64,53,54]. Similarly, the introduction of user charges at public and private health facilities has become standard practice, as has been seen in Afghanistan and southern Sudan. In the case of the former, there has been a push to announce it as the Government's official policy. An overriding concern in Iraq has been how to evacuate victims of violence from the site of an incident to the nearest emergency medical centre, an issue that was regularly raised in the media because of its huge humanitarian, social and political dimension (personal communication).

Health systems in conflict settings can, as in "normal" situations, support a healthy life, or, by their absence or ineffectiveness, undermine it and perpetuate health inequity. It is especially essential in emergencies to maintain services at two levels. Firstly, it is important to ensure an essential package of health services to all, covering areas such as maternal and child health, childhood immunization, HIV/AIDS and the provision of essential medicines for malaria, the tuberculosis directly observed treatment, short-course (DOTS) strategy, and for other common health problems. Secondly, medical services should be accessible to the victims of conflict and violence, and for emergencies that are seen in any "normal" situation by making accessible life-saving medicines (e.g. insulin, anti-hypertensive medicines), and services (e.g. emergency obstetric services).

In crisis situations, many organizations, such as ministries of health, development partners, nongovernmental organizations and private services are likely to be called upon to provide health services. Lebanon had always depended on a complex system of for-profit and not-for-profit health services, with the Ministry of Public Health largely uninvolved; nevertheless, these organizations appeared to work together well during the crisis of summer 2006 according to the civil society report. In other countries, such as Afghanistan and (southern) Sudan, as the public sector delivery systems have become progressively destroyed, nongovernmental organizations have played an increasingly prominent role in service delivery. This has started a huge debate on whether to contract out health services to nongovernmental organizations in such countries, especially in post-conflict situations. In the Region, evidence has shown that there is a place for the carefully regulated contracting out of health services, especially in the short term [102].

Chapter 6
Views and voices from civil society[1]

6.1 Afghanistan

The civil society study conducted by a research team from two nongovernmental organizations, the Social and Health Development Programme and Care of the Afghan Family, captures in qualitative terms the impact of conflict on the health and well-being of Afghans. Interviews and focus group discussions were held in Kabul from 24 February to 2 March 2007, including in-depth interviews with staff of ministries and relief workers, and focus group discussions with staff of nongovernmental organizations working directly with affected people, and with refugees and IDPs.

The following perceptions from individuals reflect their desperation with the situation in the country.

- "harm does not mean just killing, but 3 million martyred, 2 million disabled, 5 million illiterate, 5 million drug addicts and 6 million refugees in Pakistan, Islamic Republic of Iran and other countries";
- "people lost their tranquillity, dignity, family members, wealth, farmlands and houses";
- "200 families live in my village, and almost 100 residents have been injured by landmines".

Marked differences in health and well-being were noted between different areas of the country, especially between the central lowlands and the remote highland frontier districts. This was seen as a reflection of the availability of health services, with more services in north-eastern, south-eastern and southern parts of the country, and in urban areas, especially Kabul.

The major health-related problems identified by respondents include: drug addiction; mental health problems; malnutrition; sexual abuse and violence and early or forced

---

[1] Except where otherwise noted, these accounts are drawn directly from the civil society reports submitted by AHED to WHO Regional Office for the Eastern Mediterranean.

marriage and rape. They estimated that drug addiction affects almost 5 million people. Drugs can be found everywhere, and even security forces are illicitly involved in drug distribution. (Afghanistan is the world's largest producer of opium, most of which is smuggled across its borders to find ready markets in the west.) Mental health problems were estimated to affect 50% of people; respondents coined the term "continuous stress" to describe the current situation over anxiety about poverty and obtaining food, and daily fear and danger. Other problems were identified as:

- malnutrition resulting in the short height of the new generation, and people going prematurely grey and losing their teeth;
- poor access to services was reflected in reports of health services in crisis: many facilities have been destroyed, others are of low quality, and have few medicines; there is a shortage of health staff, especially females, and many staff have left the country;
- the deterioration in agriculture, irrigation systems, forests and access to fuel;
- scarcity of safe water, even in large cities;
- disruption of foodstuff transportation to remote areas;
- damage to schools, unavailability of teachers; the lack of teacher training and education for girls (boys may also be forbidden to go to school).

The consensus was that some groups were especially vulnerable because:

- the poor can not afford to flee from danger, especially those near front-line fighting in Kabul;
- youth face death or physical disability;
- women receive poorer treatment at health facilities than men, and face complications of pregnancy and sexual violence;
- children suffer from undernutrition, infectious diseases and abuse;
- refugees have no access to regular health services, except immunization during national immunization days (NIDs);
- nomads (between one fifth and one seventh of the population) and IDPs are not covered by existing health services.

Coping strategies were related to individual and family ability. Wealthier people left the country or moved to safer cities, where health and social services were better. The most wealthy migrated to the USA, Europe and other developed countries; the middle class to the Islamic Republic of Iran and Pakistan. Currently, wealthy people go to Pakistan or India for medical treatment.

6.2 Doctors for Iraq: a nongovernmental organization reporting from Iraq

The following comments on the current situation in Iraq were compiled by the nongovernmental organization Doctors for Iraq in April 2007. They reflect the comments of doctors trying to uphold their professional obligations in increasingly difficult conditions, as the conflict escalates and the boundaries between the forces involved become increasingly blurred.

The conditions that doctors and other health staff have to cope with also reflect the fears and frustrations of those who need their services: "There is no minor health problem...having an illness is a tragedy by itself, because it means suffering for the patient and his relatives".

For patients access to health services was often a problem: difficulty in accessing surviving health services because of checkpoints, road blocks, curfews and lack of transport; IDPs, especially those in remote areas, have the greatest difficulty accessing health services; and patients (and health staff) are also frustrated that health centres have insufficient medicines and equipment.

Doctors identified the groups most likely to suffer poor health during the period of conflict as:

- men, who from the beginning of the conflict became involved in fighting, later became targets for kidnapping and assassination;
- children are the "silent victims"; increasingly children and women have become victims of attacks on markets and schools;
- children and women are also suffering from a lack of access to health facilities;
- prisoners endure appalling conditions; the organization visited a government prison and recorded that scabies, diarrhoea and tuberculosis were widespread; prisoners lacked medical attention, especially those suffering from chronic diseases, such as hypertension and diabetes.

Doctors identified common health problems in Iraq, such as communicable and noncommunicable diseases and injuries, arising from the conflict. Communicable diseases are increasing, and typhoid, hepatitis A and diarrhoea are appearing in crowded areas of cities, in remote areas and among the IDP population; children suffer from diarrhoeal diseases, respiratory infections and malnutrition, mostly in remote areas and among IDPs; and doctors have started seeing diseases that they have rarely seen before, such as typhoid, hepatitis and measles.

Noncommunicable diseases include chronic illnesses, such as hypertension and diabetes mellitus, which are increasing; patients suffer because of shortage of medication, poor quality of medicines and poor case management (on problems of storing and distributing insulin, see Mansour and Wanoose, 2007 [103]). An increase in leukaemia was noted over the last year in Basra, the west of Iraq and in Baghdad.

Other health problems include drug abuse and mental illness. Drug abuse, especially among young people, is evidenced by the increasing number of people being taken to hospital as a result of an overdose. Mental illness, especially depression, is difficult to deal with because of the stigma associated with it.

Since April 2003 doctors have reported seeing new kinds of injuries from the conflict, including injuries from cluster bombs, and over the last year, an increase in multi-shell injuries (including nails) mostly on the head and chest; patients with such injuries die before reaching hospital because of severe bleeding and the lack of first aid at the scene or in the ambulance. New weapons cause suffocation and first and second degree burns; doctors in Ramadi reported two attacks with chlorine gas which killed victims and spread irritating toxic gas in the surrounding area; most victims were children. Burns units do not have the capacity to deal with these injuries.

Doctors who were interviewed were concerned about breaches of medical neutrality, in contravention of the Geneva Convention, which they considered to be undermining the whole health system. They referred to attacks on health units and arrests of health workers. In addition, they noted that ethnic and political discrimination was rife with most employees in a facility coming from the same ethnic background or sharing the same political affiliation; doctors also alleged that the militias were infiltrating the Ministry of Health and the hospitals.

The doctors interpreted the overall outcome of this situation as contributing to the breakdown of trust and confidence between patients and health providers, for example, people are afraid to go to a provider or facility associated with a different ethnic or political background, and to the mass migration of health workers from Iraq; the Ministry of Health estimates that one half of the country's doctors have fled [37].

Doctors reported the development of coping strategies to respond to the health crisis such as: doctors opening clinics in their homes rather than in commercial areas, which they see as less secure; people visiting pharmacies or a local nurse rather than a doctor; people returning to the use of natural remedies and herbs; and women returning to dependence on midwives and on delivering at home.

6.3 Resilience and social networks in the Lebanon crisis

The civil society interviews were conducted by an academic on behalf of AHED. The interviews, which took place with government officials, members of nongovernmental organizations and other key informants, need to be seen against the backdrop of the short, extremely destructive armed conflict of July–August 2006 which resulted in:

- 1 million people of a total population of 4 million fleeing their homes: 27 000 people fled the country; 735 000 people were displaced within the country; 130 000 found shelter in schools and parks and the remainder in private homes;
- 1184 civilians killed and 4059 injured [98];
- destruction of infrastructure: in the most severely affected areas 50%–70% of health facilities have been destroyed; only one third of all facilities have potable water [104]; 73 bridges and 400 miles of roads destroyed; breakdown in water, sewerage and electric power supply; more than a quarter of all health facilities badly damaged or destroyed; 350 schools destroyed; 15 000 homes destroyed, 13 000 badly damaged; bombing and closure of Beirut International Airport;
- an oil spill over 150 km of coastline;
- minefields with over one million unexploded cluster bombs [98]; for documentation of violations of human rights and international humanitarian law see 105, 106.

Comments from interviewees on access to, and quality of, goods and services during and immediately after the conflict included:

- people who stayed in their homes south of the Litani River lived in a state of siege during the hostilities; populations who moved north had better access to facilities;
- IDPs and residents south of the Litani River suffered from a lack of safe water;
- those living in schools reported problems accessing sanitation facilities;
- emergency evacuation services were hindered by the destruction of roads and bridges;
- former residents returned to the south quickly after the end of the war, presenting a challenge to emergency services, which provided food rations for two months and tents and blankets.

Features of the conflict that had an impact on health in the view of the interviewees included:

- family dislocation: the population in areas in the south under the most intense fire was just recovering from years of Israeli occupation that ended in 2000;
- unanticipated scope and intensity of destruction;
- obliteration of several towns and villages, and destruction in the southern suburbs of Beirut;

- systematic destruction of transport, water, electricity and telephone communications;
- violation of international humanitarian law and Geneva Conventions, including strikes on ambulances, hospitals and civilian convoys.

Coping strategies were expressed in terms of the "solidarity factor", shared resilience and responsibility; a sense of pride in the resistance that faced the assault: in spite of former divisions, a gritty confidence that they would pull through. Evidence from civil society sources includes:

- the reception of the majority of IDPs in homes rather than shelters; families hosted IDPs regardless of ethnic/sectarian differences;
- the ability of communities under siege in the area south of the Litani River to access loans, food, clothing and other resources left by neighbours who had fled;
- the immediate return to the devastated areas south of the Litani River, which was seen as a coping strategy;
- the importance of spirituality, especially noted were group prayers by IDPs;
- the focusing on daily needs and not being too demanding on relief workers.

People helped each other depending on their situation and abilities. The resilience, especially of the IDPs, and resourcefulness which contributed to the prevention of epidemics and psychological breakdown in the short term, was associated with prior preparation, informed by a continued awareness of the recurrence of past humanitarian disasters [107]. During the period of civil war, 1975–1992, it was also noted that civilians were determined to maintain their daily routine [108].

6.4 The Gaza Strip and the impact of the separation wall on life in the occupied Palestinian territory

The civil society report compiled by the nongovernmental organization, the Palestinian Medical Relief Society, in April 2007, draws on official reports, personal interviews and one focus group discussion. From the long report, this review focuses on the impact on health of the separation wall being built in the West Bank.

The Gaza Strip, with a population density of 3808 per km^2, one of the most crowded places on earth, and the West Bank, are both suffering acutely in the current crisis, with two thirds of the population living below the poverty line, and approximately 50% of people unemployed [99, 109]. The situation has deteriorated markedly since this report was compiled in March 2007.

The separation wall around the West Bank has worsened conditions for all Palestinians. The wall, whose construction began in June 2002, will stretch for 670 km, and will split the West Bank into five regions, separating the rest of the West Bank completely from East Jerusalem. Checkpoints and road blocks in the Gaza Strip and in the West Bank in association with the separation wall restrict movement within and between the West Bank and the Gaza Strip, preventing Palestinians from meeting family and kin, and accessing employment and social services, such as health care and education.

The construction of the wall has denied many Palestinians access to health care. Forty-one health care facilities are now isolated, with the wall almost 50% complete; 22 are in vulnerable enclaves; 23 are in government facilities, 15 are run by nongovernmental organizations, two by the United Nations Relief and Works Agency for Palestine Refugees in the Near East (UNRWA), and one is private. Of the currently isolated facilities: 36% reported that many of their patients can no longer attend; 53% received new patients who could no longer attend their former health centres; 63% reported delays in the delivery of services by their mobile and medical teams; and 55% reported difficulties in accessing medicine for chronic diseases.

Palestinian ambulances are not allowed to enter the area between the Green Line and the wall. As the International Court of Justice has declared the wall and gate system and the permits illegal, UN and nongovernmental organization staff are not applying for permits for staff, so they cannot continue mobile health services and supplementary food distribution [110,111].

Between September 2005 and the end of 2005, the combined impact of closures (checkpoints, road blocks and the wall) resulted in the death at checkpoints of 129 people denied access to hospitals, and at least 67 deliveries at checkpoints resulting in the death of 36 newborn infants and five mothers [61].

In rural areas, the proportion of deliveries taking place at home increased from 5% prior to the *intifada* to approximately 30% during the times of strict closures in 2003, primarily because women were unwilling to undergo the stressful journey to a health facility [112].

The UN General Assembly resolution (GA/10560) on 15 December 2006, to establish a register of damage arising from the construction of the wall by Israel in the occupied Palestinian territory, noted that "the damage was severe, vast and continuous" and involved "violations of the Palestinian people's freedom of movement and their right to work, to health, to education and to an adequate standard of living; as well as the displacement of Palestinian civilians from their homes and lands" [113].

The route of the wall, as officially approved by the Israeli Government, will directly affect the health of approximately 425 000 people, about one fifth of the West Bank's residents. It will affect 12 750 older people, 183 000 children aged 14 and younger, and 77 000 children under 5 years of age, who will need vaccinations. Approximately 12 750 people with disabilities will be prevented from reaching required specialized health care in central cities such as Ramallah and Jerusalem [61], and 71 clinics will be isolated, assuming that existing clinics will remain functioning.

Some specialized services for Palestinians in the Gaza Strip and the West Bank are only available in East Jerusalem, such as eye surgery, open heart surgery, oncological treatments and heart surgery for children; and hospitals in East Jerusalem have reported a drastic decline in the number of patients, jeopardizing their existence.

The completed wall will place 46% of West Bank land out of reach of Palestinians. Residents in the area between the Green Line, the internationally recognized boundary between Israel and the occupied Palestinian territory, and the wall will be especially affected as they require permits to live there and to cross into the West Bank proper [110,111,114]. The stress of negotiating all these barriers on a day-to-day basis cannot but have a serious effect on the physiological well-being of residents. Restricted mobility will increasingly affect all aspects of the life of those living in enclosed areas; access to employment, social activities, relatives and friends; and to services such as health care and schools.

6.5 Surviving in Somalia

The Somali civil society report was compiled by the nongovernmental organization, Somali Organization for Community Development Activities, in Mogadishu, in April 2007, under great difficulty because of the daily escalation of the conflict in the city. While conditions in the north-west and north-east are fairly secure, they reported that current conditions in the rest of Somalia are dire after 16 years of civil conflict.

- There is no effective government or infrastructure, or regional health authorities.
- Over 1 million civilians have fled the country and 0.5 million are in IDP camps.
- Unarmed civilians are suffering most acutely, with at least six civilians being killed every day and many more injured, by sniper fire and unexploded combat devices.
- Droughts, floods and the Indian Ocean tsunami in 2004 have affected health, resulting in epidemics of diarrhoea and cholera.
- Free education has disappeared.
- People with mental health disorders wander around urban centres.
- People smuggling across the Arabian Sea to Yemen continues, with many fatalities en route [115].
- State health services collapsed when the government ceased to exist in January 1991; all government hospitals in Somalia, especially in Mogadishu, were looted and destroyed. Currently, some private hospitals and clinics have been established, but only the upper class business people can afford them; refugees, IDPs, people with physical disabilities, orphans, street people and the unemployed cannot afford health

care; some hospitals offer inexpensive services but transport costs are too high for disadvantaged people to reach them.

In Mogadishu, the capital, the focus of the current fighting, as of April 2007: almost a quarter of the city's 1.5 million people are moving out of the city; cheap municipal water and electricity services have collapsed and bore-holes and generators are beyond the reach of all but the rich; there is no state authority to control water quality; rubbish collection and sanitation services have disappeared; and rubbish mountains represent a hazard to health.

Cholera was confirmed in Mogadishu in March 2007. The outbreak was related to the complete breakdown of health and water systems, continued fighting and population displacement. The usual responses to the outbreak, such as supplying clean water and oral rehydration therapy, were not available [116].

Coping strategies discussed in the civil society report include the preservation of clan and subclan organizations which provide people with a social identity and support network and the establishment of community-based organizations to help those in need.

6.6 Darfur

The Darfurian civil society interviews were conducted by AHED. Since 2003, Darfur, in western Sudan, has suffered extensive civil conflict. This has resulted in the destruction of the homes, villages and livelihoods of many Darfurians. Major health problems result from a lack of clean water and adequate housing; northern Darfur, which is mainly desert, is most seriously affected by lack of water. By mid-2006, 200 000 Darfurians had died, mostly from conflict-related diseases and malnutrition, and 2 million had been forced from their homes. The conflict has now spread to neighbouring Chad [3,26].

Civilian respondents from Darfur noted that women suffer from rape and harassment, and also malnutrition which contributes to the death of their children. Children suffer from malnutrition, which is most acute during the rainy season, and trauma because of bombardment, militia raids and the killing of family members. Attacks by armed groups on aid workers have caused a suspension of some aid activities.

Aid organizations responded to the crisis by providing emergency surgery, basic health care, antenatal and postnatal care, rehabilitation for rape victims and therapeutic and supplementary feeding during peaks of malnutrition. However, education has been neglected.

Coping strategies include attempts by IDPs to organize themselves into social groups based on their tribes. However, most IDPs are now politicized, as armed groups emerged which were tribally based making them vulnerable to attack by other groups in the camps.

Chapter 7
Addressing social determinants and protecting health in conflicts: Everybody's business

7.1 Strategies to protect health through a social determinants approach

In the face of immense challenges and in the absence of lack of adherence to standard guidelines to protect health, addressing the social determinants of health in conflict settings is everybody's business—citizens, local community-based organizations, international nongovernmental organizations, the media and academia, governments, development partners and indeed global players and powers.

Given the often intractable nature of conflicts, many become chronic over time, with major implications for all aspects of the lives and health of the people who are forced to live in the arduous circumstances created by conflict. In some ways, such conflicts, because of their malignant character, can be likened to cancers that attack the human body. There are no standard prescriptions and each conflict situation requires its own set of interventions. As has been the case with cancers, at least in the past, most interventions to tackle conflicts have remained palliative and few have attacked the root cause. Perhaps the main difference is that the suffering due to cancers is largely due to lack of technological development and that due to conflicts is due to lack of political will and commitment.

Strategies to protect health through a social determinants approach are either directed at the intermediate determinants, which focus on the individual, family and community level, or at the structural determinants, which focus on the national, regional and global level to address the root of the problem. Strategies to tackle the intermediate determinants can be viewed as micro-strategies, and strategies to tackle the structural determinants as macro-strategies, without being judgemental of the importance of either (Box 3). Perhaps not surprisingly, there is far more information about the micro-strategies adopted by individuals and communities, assisted by civil societies, to cope with some of the most extraordinary circumstances that they have to confront than there is about macro-strategies. Macro-strategies to address the structural determinants and the global distribution of power and resources are discussed further in Chapter 8.

> **Box 3. Strategies at the micro-level: addressing intermediate determinants**
> - Strengthen family and community networks for sustainable, healthy development, especially through work with civil society.
> - Strengthen capabilities for sustainable development through the creation of employment and livelihood initiatives, and the provision of education, housing and safe water and sanitation.
> - Reconstruct and maintain essential health services, working with partners and strengthening the role of ministries of health.

7.2 Interventions at the individual, family and community levels

A number of promising responses to conflict, which help to ameliorate the dire conditions described in this publication, are identified here. Because of the orientation of this publication, they are based on a bottom-up rather than top-down view of crises. However, most of these activities can best be described as promising rather than proved. Serious evaluations of relief efforts (including those of nongovernmental organizations) that could provide evidence for "best practices" to ameliorate the impact of conflict on civilian populations are rare. These tentative beginnings will, it is hoped, respond to the need for locally-adapted, evidence-based examples that would both deal with the immediate crisis and assist in the transition to longer term development [47].

Many countries in crisis depend on funding provided by bilateral agencies and multilateral organizations to maintain or restore health systems which have been shattered by the crisis. International agencies often turn to international, and especially locally-based, nongovernmental organizations to deliver health services, sometimes on a contractual basis. Nongovernmental organizations working in local settings are thus able to expand existing services or to provide new ones. However, they, and all other partners involved in health and welfare interventions in a crisis setting, need to be able to move from a crisis mode towards more sustainable, long-term programmes that will support a range of related activities.

Working at the individual, family and community levels provides opportunities and challenges for tackling the serious problem of mental health. A psychosocial approach in a conflict setting should go beyond the individual to the wider social setting within which loss is experienced. This approach has added value for all community members, as it deals with mental health problems through social and community-based activities designed to increase the resilience of the population, provide support for the whole family, and increase community solidarity [20,21,117]. Nongovernmental organizations are ideally suited to incorporate these approaches into their work in conflict settings.

The Palestinian Medical Relief Society supports a programme for targeted populations living in extreme poverty and suffering from a lack of food and economic resources due to closures and the restricted mobility of people and goods. The Society mobilizes its resources to reach those living in the most remote, isolated and poor regions, which are not being provided with services from the national authority or other organizations. It does not rely only on food provision to tackle malnutrition, as this approach has created problems of dependency. In order to tackle malnutrition and anaemia in a comprehensive manner, the programme first screened affected families and provided medical treatment and vitamins. It then provided job creation activities for target households and individuals living below the poverty line, paying them for their labour. Job creation programmes focused on developing community assets by building schools, clinics and kindergartens. Support for female-headed households was also provided, working with organizations already active in this field. The Palestinian Medical Relief Society provided individuals with sheep and goats, a source of milk and cheese for households, a valuable source of nutrition for the household. It also assisted women to enter the market and sell their products [112].

The Gaza Community Mental Health Programme began in 1990. During the second *intifada* the conflict rapidly escalated and there was a growing need for mental health assistance as a result of the increased prevalence of mental disorders among the population increasingly exposed to trauma, violence and torture. These acts of violence disturbed family members and entire communities, neighbourhoods, schools and children. A new approach to mental health, with a greater community orientation that directly addressed dysfunctions in the social environment was identified, moving away from the institutional therapeutic approaches then available through the Ministry of Health. Human rights considerations for community members were the reference points for organizing the programme and for delivering services. Because violence is felt at all levels in the community, the programme aims to simultaneously address many sectors of the society. It aims to give tools to the community to enable it to face future problems in the long term. The programme works with the Ministry of Health and UNRWA to deliver complementary services, meeting regularly to assess and coordinate crisis interventions. Thirty per cent of the effort has focused on delivering clinical services for people in need. Training and research engage up to 70% of the programme, which is seen as essential for gathering evidence and for capacity-building [67,68,89,112].

Protection against sexual violence in Darfur has focused on listening to women, female empowerment and providing protection for risky activities. Responding to concerns voiced in the civil society report about sexual violence, local nongovernmental organizations can and do support individual and small group activities, but must have the support of international agencies with a responsibility to maintain security and human rights.

Women's centres provide female victims of sexual violence with resources, support and referral. Women share their individual stories, recognizing that where rape is used as a weapon of war the experience is a collective one. By providing a safe space for women to build trust, share experiences and rest from the tasks of daily survival, such centres provide a source of empowerment to women [118]. In response to sexual violence, IDPs called for: increased prevention and response to sexual and gender-based violence; community-based policing based on dialogue with IDPs; health facilities that offer privacy to women, and are able to treat them for fistula; and birth attendants and community leaders trained to deal with the health and emotional needs of survivors of sexual violence [119,120].

Women in Darfur are in danger of being raped while collecting firewood, both for their own use or to sell. Solutions attempted included firewood patrols and the use of efficient stoves and/or alternative fuels. Firewood patrols could protect women outside the camps, however, they have often been ineffective as a result of the difficulty of communication between the women and the civilian police or troops assigned to protect them. The use of fuel efficient stoves and/or alternative fuels would obviate the need for women to go outside the camp to collect firewood [24].

7.3 Cooperation to improve health care and access to care

Collaboration between the many actors responsible for health care in crisis is essential. The WHO Regional Office for the Eastern Mediterranean has been working in conflict-affected countries to ensure the continuation of basic health services, in cooperation with other partners, and undertakes a major coordinating role in the health sector. In a conflict setting it is essential to support the role of the ministries of health, and to support their future role as a regulatory agency, as well as a provider of basic health services. Often, ministries of health have been fatally weakened and, by default, much care is provided by voluntary, non-profit organizations. Ministries of health have a vital role to play in regulating and managing the activities of nongovernmental organizations, rationalizing the provision over all geographic areas and ensuring equitable access.

In Afghanistan, the seriously under-resourced Ministry of Public Health embarked on a programme to contract out a Basic Package of Health Services to nongovernmental organizations, which were already providing most of the health care in the country. Although these services, which may be provided through existing ministry facilities, resulted in a positive improvement in access to basic health services, the short-term contracts fostered a short-term "quick fix" view of the task. Such contracts need to be carefully managed and monitored in the interests of long-term sustainability. Strengthening the essential management and oversight functions of the Ministry will improve the Ministry's ability to influence policy-makers and deliver a sustainable and equitable service delivery system in more peaceful times [121].

Where many health facilities have been destroyed or severely damaged, and many health staff have fled, it is essential to rebuild and refurbish facilities and ensure that they are staffed by trained health workers. Regional Office technical support to nurses, midwives and other cadres, in collaboration with partners, includes support for institutes of health sciences and nursing/midwifery in Somalia, Afghanistan and Sudan, plans of action on nursing and midwifery in Iraq and Somalia, and curriculum development in Afghanistan and Somalia.

In Somalia, the Regional Office is supporting collaborative programmes to strengthen nursing schools to provide nurses and midwives for all three zones of Somalia: in Bossaso, Mogadishu, and Garawe and at the Institute of Health Sciences in Hargeisa. The need for such services was illustrated by a May 2007 assessment in the Sanaag Region which found that most health posts were closed except for those run by the Somali Red Crescent Society; the last training of trained birth attendants took place 5 years ago; and all deliveries took place at home with unskilled birth attendants [122]. In Afghanistan, technical support is being provided to institutes of health sciences and the community midwifery programme. Currently, there is a serious shortage of female health workers due to security problems and restrictions on women's education and work; as of July 2006, 90% of trainee nurses were male [123].

The north-west zone of Somalia is making an attempt to rebuild the health system following widespread destruction of health facilities and mass migration or death of health workers. International linkages, specifically with institutions in the United Kingdom, support rebuilding facilities, staffing and especially professional education [124]. This effort is quoted as a "rare success story of post-conflict reconstruction" [125].

In the West Bank areas affected by the separation wall, as of early 2005 (before the crisis of 2006), mobile clinics operated jointly by the Ministry of Health and UNRWA provided the full package of primary health care services, including vaccination, antenatal care and care for chronically-ill people. These clinics were part of the emergency response project and became more important after the extension of closures and the construction of the separation wall. In early 2005, these clinics served more than 26 000 beneficiaries in 135 remote locations, reducing the percentage of the population not receiving health care from 70% to 50%. Funds and coordination provided by the European Union and European Commission Humanitarian Office (ECHO) were crucial in supporting this system of mobile clinics. According to the Palestinian civil society report: "Mobile clinics represent a success story in coordination, resource use and human intention, as mobile clinic staff put their lives at risk to serve the Palestinian population and provide it with the opportunity to live a healthy life."

In Afghanistan, the Ministry of Public Health is responding to particular health problems. Prompted in part by the preliminary results of the 1999–2002 reproductive age mortality study, the Ministry identified a reduction in maternal mortality as a major objective [54].

In Lebanon, regular Ministry of Public Health services continued to be provided during the 2006 conflict, in extremely difficult circumstances, and no major disease outbreaks were recorded. Interventions that helped to mitigate the impact of the conflict on health included collaborative activities and the expanding role of nongovernmental organizations. As noted in the civil society report, the Ministries of Public Health and Social Affairs provided full coverage of medical care for casualties irrespective of nationality, including ambulatory services, hospitalization, prostheses and rehabilitation. Emergency services were jointly managed by the private sector, nongovernmental organizations, hospital syndicates, medical suppliers, the Lebanese Red Cross and Red Crescent (with international partners), civil defence and the army. Two clusters were established; one for hospital services and one for primary health care. With many new nongovernmental organizations established, the activities of these organization have included: directly providing health care; following IDPs back to their villages and involving local residents in relief operations; supporting women in establishing small enterprises; working with youth in the areas of entertainment, conducting awareness-raising on behavioural issues and promoting sport.

Chapter 8
Tackling the root causes

Conflicts, especially in the Region, are not one-off events. They are often chronic, lasting for years. Their origin and perpetuation are closely tied to a world system that has grown more complex since 1945. The morbidity and mortality that is indirectly associated with conflict is difficult to identify and to disentangle from morbidity and mortality due to other underlying causes of poor health. This is especially the case in countries of the Region which have long records of poor health outcomes due to the combined impact of conflict, poverty and ineffective health systems.

Conflict can damage the health of people in various ways. It may directly affect physical and mental health, and it may disrupt health systems and damage infrastructure that affects health, such as water supplies or sanitation services. The impact of a crisis on health will depend on local circumstances; in a low-income country a crisis may destroy the potential for an improvement in health, or it may cause the health services of a formerly middle-income country to plunge into chaos. Although some of the social determinants of health in conflict settings may not necessarily be different from those in non-conflict settings, they reflect and further reinforce existing inequalities and the

---

Box 4. Strategies at the macro-level: addressing structural determinants

- Conflict transformation and "Health as a bridge for peace" can be used as platforms for spreading peace and well-being in the Region, and dialogue within and between countries.
- Regional and global forums such as the League of Arab States, the European Commission, the Group of Eight (G8), and the United Nations should guarantee to protect the health of people living in countries under occupation or civil strife.
- The League of Arab States may have a special role to play in many countries through promotion of human rights, democracy and good governance.
- WHO can play a role in providing evidence on the impact of conflicts on health in the Region and beyond.
- Organizations from countries of occupying forces which promote human rights and protect health should be implored to raise their voices on behalf of vulnerable populations.

vulnerability of those who are disadvantaged because of poverty, marginalization and discrimination.

The WHO Regional Office for the Eastern Mediterranean, individual countries in the Region and civil society partners expressed concerns that the particular social determinants of health associated with conflicts in the Region should be identified and explored. As a result of these concerns the Commission on Social Determinants of Health requested a review from the Region and through this review three social determinants that have a bearing on health and which are peculiar to a conflict setting were identified: loss of human rights, breaches of medical neutrality and progression from stress to distress and disease. As noted in Chapter 1, the Commission on Social Determinants of Health identifies several ways of looking at social determinants. The structural determinants of health in conflict settings include the broad economic, cultural, historical, environmental and "political" determinants of health at the country and global level. These affect power relationships that determine the distribution of power, prestige and resources globally and within a particular country or society, including those needed to maintain health and social well-being.

The structural determinants are reflected in the intermediate, and strictly more "social" determinants, the conditions in which people live which affect their health status. The loss of human rights is the first and most important of the major structural determinants in conflict settings. The second major structural determinant, breaches of medical neutrality, is especially relevant for the right to health care, as combatants attempt to weaken the resistance of civilians by deliberately depriving them of access to care, especially at the times when they most need it. They are violations of the Fourth Geneva Convention, Article 18 [29].

Armed conflict results in life settings that produce high levels of mortality, disability and morbidity (physical as well as mental), directly or indirectly resulting from the conflict, when compared to health outcomes in otherwise comparable non-conflict settings. From a social determinants and public health perspective, it is essential to link together, both conceptually and in practice, the strategies that are needed to work at the different levels: local, regional and national (see Box 4 for macro-level strategies).

One way of addressing the structural determinants at national level is to look at the concept of conflict transformation, as an innovative approach to mitigate the health impact of armed conflict. It starts from the understanding that "conflicts are embedded in relations at the individual, interpersonal, organizational, community and international levels, and include psychological, sociocultural, spiritual, political, historical and economic dimensions" [126]. Conflict transformation incorporates an appreciation of the value of participation, inclusiveness, empowerment, social justice and healing at the community level, as well as at regional and national levels. This approach recognizes the loss felt by people caught in the tragedy of conflict. Above all, it identifies the importance of dialogue and openness, and the need for participants in dialogue to be freed from thinking strictly within the framework of their own interests and oppositional positions.

At national level dialogue needs to be initiated to recognize the major challenges that are being faced, such as governance, social and economic inequity, low education levels, human rights and foreign occupation. Health can be a bridge for peace, a way of beginning a transformational dialogue about such issues. Although public debate about health is rare in most countries of the Region, getting the social and political issues underlying health problems on to the agenda could have positive effects on the Region's current socioeconomic–political dilemma. The increasing reach of global health organizations can have a positive impact only if they support a consensus on the value of primary health care to strengthen health systems in both stable and conflict-affected areas. The increasing range and scope of international organizations, the recognition of civil society as a "voice" of the people, and of the human rights agenda and international humanitarian law can have a positive impact. They present opportunities for people and organizations within the Region to open up dialogue, with external and internal actors, about the problems faced by fragile countries, such as lack of arms control, prejudicial terms of trade, and food and resource scarcity, all of which exacerbate armed conflict.

There is a need to leverage the potential of regional and global forums such as the League of Arab States, the European Commission, the Group of Eight (G8) and the United Nations, to promote and protect the health of populations living in countries under occupation or civil strife. The League of Arab States may have a special role to play in many countries through the promotion of human rights, democracy and good governance. Development agencies, especially agencies such as WHO which has a special mandate to respond to health needs in crisis settings, should work together to provide health services. They can also act as advocates, with other global institutions, to use health as a bridge for peace in the world. The mandate of WHO to provide health data extends to presenting evidence on the impact of conflicts on health; this is essential advocacy material that is needed to spur action by all partners on addressing health and well-being in conflict-affected countries. There are also a large number of organizations from countries of occupation forces which support the promotion of civil liberties and human rights, and the protection of health not just for their own citizens, but equally, for vulnerable populations across the globe; their potential needs to be harnessed.

As noted in Chapter 7, collaboration between the many actors responsible for health care in crisis is essential. Ministries of health in countries in conflict are weakened and care may be provided by voluntary, non-profit organizations. The role of ministries of health in regulating and managing the activities of nongovernmental organizations, rationalizing the provision of health services in all geographic areas and in ensuring equitable access is vital.

All civil society reports noted the development of coping strategies to respond to conflict situations and the creation of social and community-based activities designed to increase the resilience of populations, provide support for families and increase community solidarity. Although the coping strategies developed by civilians in conflict vary, maintaining and strengthening social networks in a changed or new setting can be a key to maintaining mental and physical health. Conflict and its attendant trauma often require that individuals undertake new roles and these roles may strengthen individuals' ability to cope in stressful situations. Individuals and communities can adapt to adversity and may even thrive in spite of it. Solidarity, shared resilience and a sense of pride in resistance are often shared by communities in conflict settings as they become active participants in social processes rather than passive observers. These qualities provide hope for a positive future in terms of a recognition of characteristics that promote positive adaptation and of resilience as an asset for future health development.

References

1. Krug EG et al. *World report on violence and health*. Geneva, World Health Organization, 2002 (http://www.who.int/violence_injury_prevention/violence/world_report/en/full_en.pdf, accessed 12 November 2007).

2. Office of the Spokesperson for the Secretary-General. Secretary-General's address at the Truman Presidential Museum and Library, December 2006 (http://www.un.org/appa/sg/sgatats.asp? Nid+2357, accessed 28 February 2008.)

3. Grono N. Briefing—Darfur: the international community's failure to protect. *African Affairs*, 2006, 105 (421):621–631. The author is affiliated with the International Crisis Group, an independent nongovernmental organization based in Brussels; www.crisisgroup.org/.

4. Commission on Social Determinants of Health. *Achieving health equity: from root causes to fair outcomes: interim statement*. Commission on Social Determinants of Health. Geneva, World Health Organization, 2007 (http://www.who.int/social_determinants/resources/interim_statement/en/index.html, accessed November 5, 2007).

5. Braveman P, Gruskin S. Defining equity in health. *Journal of Epidemiology and Community Health*, 2003, 57(4):254–8.

6. Sen A. Elements of a theory of human rights. *Philosophy and Public Affairs*, 2004, 32(4):315–356.

7. Commission on Social Determinants of Health. *A conceptual framework for action on the social determinants of health*; discussion paper for the Commission on Social Determinants of Health, Draft, April 2007. Geneva, World Health Organization, 2007. (see also http://www.who.int/social_determinants/knowledge_networks/en/index.htm, accessed October 28, 2007).

8. Uppsala University. Department of Peace and Conflict Research. Uppsala, Sweden, 2007 (http://www.pcr.uu.se/database/definitions_all.htm, accessed 5 November 2007).

9. International Committee of the Red Cross. Occupied territory – the legal issues, 2007 (http://www.icrc.org/Web/Eng/siteeng0.nsf/htmlall/section_ihl_occupied_territory?OpenDocument, accessed 5 November 2007).

10. Ugalde A et al. The health costs of war: can they be measured? Lessons from El Salvador. *British Medical Journal*, 2000, 321(7254):169–72.

11. Bostoen K et al. Methods for health surveys in difficulty settings; charting progress, moving forward. *Emerging Themes in Epidemiology*, 2007, 4:14.

12. Burnham G et al. Mortality after the 2003 invasion of Iraq: a cross-sectional cluster sample survey. *The Lancet*, 2006, 368(9545):1421–8.

13. Bohannon J. Iraqi death estimates called too high; methods faulted. *Science*, 314:396–7 and letters *Science*, 2006, 314:1241.

14. Boseley S. *UK scientists attack Lancet study over death toll*. The Guardian (UK), 24 October 2006 (http://www.guardian.co.uk/international/story/0,1929817,00.html, accessed 1 November 2007).

15. Keiger D. The number. *Johns Hopkins Magazine*, 2007, 59(1).

16. Horton R. *A monstrous war crime: with more than 650,00 civilians dead in Iraq, our government must take responsibility for its lies*, The Guardian (UK), 28 March 2007 (http://www.guardian.co.uk/Iraq/Story/0,2044345,00.html accessed 1 November 2007).

17. Stein DJ et al. Post-traumatic stress disorder: medicine and politics. *The Lancet*, 2007, 369(9556):139–144.

18. Summerfield D. The invention of post-traumatic stress disorder and the social usefulness of a psychiatric category. *British Medical Journal*, 2001, 322 (7278):95–98.

19. Summerfield D. War and mental health: a brief overview. *British Medical Journal*, 2000, 321(7255):232–5.

20. Murray A. Assessing psychosocial distress – which lens? *Humanitarian Exchange* (Humanitarian Practice Network, Overseas Development Institute, UK), 2006, 36:32–35.

21. Hundt GL et al. Advocating multi-disciplinarity in studying complex emergencies: the limitations of the psychological approach to understanding how young people cope with prolonged conflict in Gaza. *Journal of Biosocial Science*, 2004, 36(4):417–31.

22. De Jong JTVM, Komproe IH. Closing the gap between psychiatric epidemiology and mental health in post-conflict situations. *The Lancet*, 2002, 359 (9540):1793–4.

23. United Nations Population Fund and WHO. *Methods and systems for the assessment and monitoring of sexual violence and exploitation in conflict situations*, December 15–16 2005, New York City, Social Science Research Council (http://www.ssrc.org/programs/HIV/publications/SVE_Report.pdf, accessed 5 November 2007).

24. Patrick E. Sexual violence and firwood collection in Darfur. *Forced Migration Review*, 2007, 27:40–41.

25. Chourou B. *Promoting human security: Ethical, normative and educational frameworks in the Arab states.* SHS/FPH/PHS/2005/PI/H/2. Paris, United Nations Educational, Scientific and Cultural Organization, 2005.

26. De Waal A. Who are the Darfurians? Arab and African identities, violence and external engagement. *African Affairs*, 2005, 104(415):181–205.

27. Abdel-Latif O. *The Shia-Sunni Divide: Myths and Reality.* Al-Ahram Weekly (Cairo), 1–7 March, 2007 (http://www.carnegieendowment.org/publications/index.cfm?fa=viewandid=19047andprog=zgpandproj=zdrl,zme, accessed 20 August 2007).

28. Stoddard A et al. *Providing aid in insecure environments: trends in policy and operations.* Humanitarian Policy Group Report 23. September 2006. Overseas Development Institute, United Kingdom, 2006.

29. International Committee of the Red Cross. International Humanitarian Law - Treaties and Documents, 2007 (http://www.icrc.org/ihl, accessed 5 November 2007).

30. Afghanistan Independent Human Rights Commission. *Violations of international humanitarian law in Afghanistan: Practices of concern and example cases.* Kabul, 2007 (http://www.aihrc.org.af/IHL_practices_and_examples_final_Coalition_Violation.pdf accessed 1 November 20007).

31. Vass A. Peace through health: This new movement needs evidence, not just ideology. *British Medical Journal*, 2001, 323(7320):1020.

32. MacQueen G, Santa-Barbara J. Peace building through health initiatives. *British Medical Journal*, 2000, 321:293–6 (http://www.humanities.mcmaster.ca/peace-health, accessed 11 June 2007).

33. WHO. *Health as a bridge for peace-humanitarian ceasefires project*, May 2001 http://www.who.int/hac/techguidance/hbp/cease_fires/en/index.html, accessed 8 October 2008).

34. UN High Commission for Refugees. *Protecting the world's most vulnerable people*, 2007 (http://www.unhcr.org/protect.html, accessed 30 April 2007).

35. UN High Commission for Refugees. News story, 2 April 2007 (http://www.unhcr.org/news/NEWS/4610f0d04.html, accessed 4 April 2007).

36. Al-Adhami M. *Refugees or angry citizens.* Al-Ahram Weekly (Cairo), 29 March–4 April, 2007, p. 6 (http://www.weekly.ahram.org.eg/2007/838/re2.htm, accessed 11 November 2007).

37. International Committee of the Red Cross. *Civilians without protection: the ever worsening humanitarian crisis in Iraq.* Released by International Committee of the Red Cross, Geneva, 11 April, 2007 (http://www.icrc.org/Web/eng/siteeng0.nsf/htmlall/iraq-report-110407/$File/Iraq-report-icrc.pdf, accessed 29 October 2007).

38. UNRWA. *Registered refugees, 31 December 2006*, 2007 (http://www.un.org.unrwa/publications.index.html, accessed 1 November 2007).

39. Poureslami IM et al. Sociocultural, environmental, and health challenges facing women and children living near the borders between Afghanistan, Iran, and Pakistan (AIP Region). *Medscape General Medicine* (MedGenMed), 2004, 6(3):51.

40. Roberts L et al. Mortality before and after the 2003 invasion of Iraq: cluster sample survey. *The Lancet*, 2004, 364(9448):1857–64.

41. Iraq Family Health Survey Study Group. Violence-related mortality in Iraq from 2002 to 2006. *The New England Journal of Medicine*, 31 January, 2008, 358:484–493.

42. Depoortere E et al. Violence and mortality in West Darfur, Sudan (2003–2004); epidemiological evidence from four surveys. *The Lancet*, 2004, 364:1315–20.

43. Grandesso F et al. Mortality and malnutrition among populations living in South Darfur, Sudan; Results of 3 surveys, September 2004. *Journal of the American Medical Association*, 2005, 293(12):1490–4.

44. Human Rights Watch. *The human cost: the consequences of insurgent attacks in Afghanistan*. Vol 19, No 6 (C), 2007 (http://www.hrw.org/reports/2007/afghanistan0407/, accessed 11 November 2007).

45. Palestinian Central Bureau of Statistics. Reporting injuries due to enemy fire, from the Palestine Red Crescent Society, 2007 (http://www.pcbs.gov.ps/Portals/_pcbs/intifada/a5d48153-b796-43ba-830d-f4d4e2a360b0.htm, accessed 16 July 2007).

46. Biluka OO et al. Death and injury from landmines and unexploded ordnance in Afghanistan. *Journal of the American Medical Association*, 2003, 290(5):650–53.

47. Moss WJ et al. Child health in complex emergencies. *Bulletin of the World Health Organization*, 2006, 84(1):58–64.

48. El-Bayoumi E. *Emissaries of mass destruction*. Al Ahram Weekly (Cairo). 25–31 January 2007, p. 13, 2007 (http://www.weekly.ahram.org.eg/2007/829/op56.htm, accessed 1 November 2007).

49. United Nations. UN General Assembly. Report of the United Nations High Commissioner for Human Rights on the follow-up to the report of the Commission of Inquiry on Lebanon, 4 June 2007 (http://daccessdds.un.org/doc/UNDOC/GEN/GO7/127/28/PDFGO712728.pdf?OpenElement, accessed 8 October 2007).

50. Ascherio A et al. Effect of the Gulf War on infant and child mortality in Iraq. *New England Journal of Medicine*, 1992, 327(13):931–6.

51. Assefa F et al. Malnutrition and mortality in Kohistan District, Afghanistan, April 2001. *Journal of the American Medical Association*, 2001, 286(21):2723–28.

52. WHO Regional Office for the Eastern Mediterranean. *Demographic, social and health indicators for countries of the Eastern Mediterranean 2006* (WHO-EM/HST/203/E), 2007.

53. Bartlett LA et al. Where giving birth is a forecast of death: maternal mortality in four districts of Afghanistan, 1999–2002. *The Lancet*, 2005, 365(9462):864–870.

54. Smith JM, Burnham G. Conceiving and dying in Afghanistan. *The Lancet*, 2005, 365(9462):827–8.

55. Amowitz LL et al. Maternal mortality in Herat Province, Afghanistan, in 2002: an indicator of women's human rights. *Journal of the American Medical Association*, 2002, 288(10):1284–91.

56. WHO. Statistical Information System (WHOSIS). Core health indicators, 2007 (http://www.who.int/whosis/database/core/core_select.cfm, accessed 5 November 2007).

57. *Human development report 2000; human rights and human development*. New York, United Nations Development Programme, 2000.

58. Hunt P. *The human right to the highest attainable standard of health: new opportunities and challenges*. Transactions of the Royal Society of Tropical Medicine and Hygiene, 2006, 100:603–7. Paul Hunt is the UN Special Rapporteur on the right to the highest attainable standard of health.

59. de Beldar B. Pity the sick of Iraq, Al-Ahram Weekly (Cairo), 5–11 April 2007, p. 10, 2007 (http://www.weekly.ahram.org.eg/2007/839/re10.htm, accessed 1 November 2007).

60. Sheibani BIM et al. Iraq lacks facilities and expertise in emergency medicine. *British Medical Journal*, 2006, 33(7573):847.

61. Palestine Ministry of Health. *Annual report 2005*. Chapter VIII, Al Aqsa Intifada, 28/09/2000–31/12/2005. Ramallah, occupied Palestinian territory, 2006.

62. Iraq. *Emergency Public Health Assistance Programme for Iraq*. Ministry of Health and WHO Iraq, 2005 (Funded by UNDG ITF).

63. Association of Iraqi Psychologists. *The psychological effects of war on Iraqis*. January 2007. Report in IRIN (UN Office for the Coordination of Humanitarian Affairs), 11 April 2007 (http://www.irinnews.org/report.aspx?reportid=69266.htm, accessed 11 November 2007).

64. Cardozo BL et al. Mental health, social functioning, and disability in postwar Afghanistan. *Journal of the American Medical Association*, 2004, 292(5):575–84.

65. Cardozo BL et al. Report from the CDC: mental health of women in postwar Afghanistan. *Journal of Women's Health*, 2005, 14(4):285–93.

66. Razokhi A et al. Mental health of Iraqi children. *The Lancet*, 2006, 368:838–9.

67. Qouta S et al. Prevalence and determinants of PTSD among Palestinian children exposed to military violence. *European Child and Adolescent Psychiatry*, 2003, 12(6):265–72.

68. Qouta S, Odeb J. The impact of conflict on children: the occupied Palestinian territory experience. *Journal of Ambulatory Care Management*, 2005, 28(1):75–9 (abstract only).

69. Thabet AA et al. Emotional problems in Palestinian children living in a war zone: a cross-sectional study. *The Lancet*, 2002, 359(9320):1801–4.

70. Al-Krenawi A et al. Psychological symptomatology among Palestinian male and female adolescents living under political violence. *Community Mental Health Journal*, 2007, 43(1):49–56.

71. Giacaman R et al. Quality of life in the Palestinian context: an inquiry in war-like conditions. *Health Policy*, 2007, 81:68–84.

72. Giacaman R et al. Individual and collective exposure to political violence: Palestinian adolescents coping with conflict. *European Journal of Public Health*, 2007, 17(4):361–368.

73. Zwi AB et al. Child health in armed conflict: time to rethink. *The Lancet*, 2006, 367:1886–8.

74. West H. Girls with guns: Narrating the experience of war of Frelimo's 'female detachment.' *Anthropological Quarterly*, 2000, 73(4):180–195.

75. Miller K.E. Research and intervention with internally displaced and refugee children. *Peace and Conflict: Journal of Peace Psychology*, 1998, 4(4):365–379.

76. UNICEF. *Nearly one million children malnourished in Iraq says UNICEF*. 26 November 1997 (http://www.unicef.org/newsline/97pr60.htm, accessed 15 April 2007).

77. Multiple Indicator Cluster Survey. Monitoring the situation of children and women: Findings from Iraq, 2006. Central Statistical Organization, Iraq, and UNICEF, 2007.

78. Multiple Indicator Cluster Survey. Multiple Indicator Cluster Survey 2000: Detailed report. Baghdad, December 2001. Central Statistical Organization, Iraq, and UNICEF, 2001.

79. UNICEF. Nutritional status survey of under five children in Baghdad–Iraq: 29 April–3 May 2003. Baghdad, Nutritional Research Institute, Ministry of Health and UNICEF, 2003.

80. *Community-based management of severe acute malnutrition*. A joint statement. WHO, UNICEF, World Food Programme, UN System Standing Committee on Nutrition, 2007 (http://www.who.int/child-adolescent-health/New_Publications/CHILD_HEALTH/Severe_Acute_Malnutrition_en.pdf, accessed 2 December 2007).

81. Federal Ministry of Health of the Government of Sudan and WHO. *Weekly Morbidity and Mortality Bulletin* (Darfur), 20–26 January 2007 (http://www.emro.who.int/Sudan/Media/PDF/WMMB_week4_07.pdf, accessed 5 November 2007).

82. Collins S et al. Management of severe acute malnutrition in children. *The Lancet*, 2006, 368:1992–2000. See also: (http://www.validinternational.org/, accessed 5 November 2007).

83. *Report on health conditions in the occupied Palestinian territory.* Regional Committee for the Eastern Mediterranean. 53rd session, Agenda item 18(a). EM/RC53/INF.DOC.11. August 2006. Cairo, WHO Regional Office for the Eastern Mediterranean, 2006 (http://www.who.int/entity/social_determinants/resources/conflicts_and_sdh_07.pdf, accessed 8 October 2008).

84. Human Rights Watch. *Rebel abuses*, 2004 (http://www.hrw.org/backgrounder/africa/darfur1104/7.htm, accessed 30 April 2007).

85. UNICEF. UNICEF News item: *James Nesbitt meets former child soldiers in southern Sudan*, 30 April 2007 (http://www.unicef.org.uk/press/news_detail.asp?news_id=942.htm, accessed 30 April 2007).

86. Hart J. Saving children: What role for anthropology? *Anthropology Today*, 2006, 22(1):5–8.

87. Palestinian Central Bureau of Statistics. Reporting deaths due to enemy fire, from the Palestine Red Cross Society, 2007 (http://www.pcbs.gov.ps/Portals/_pcbs/intifada/93b5ac0b-f061-455a-bd93-0337c0f63d, accessed 25 October 2007).

88. Chatty D, Hundt G. *Lessons learned report: children and adolescents in Palestinian households: living with the effects of prolonged conflict and forced migration.* 2nd printing, March 2002. Oxford University, Refugee Studies Centre, 2002 (htpp://www.unesdoc.unesco.org/images/0015/001511/151144e.pdf, accessed 5 November 2007).

89. Punamaki RL et al. The role of peritraumatic dissociation and gender in the association between trauma and mental health in a Palestinian community sample. *American Journal of Psychiatry*, 2005, 162(3):545–51.

90. Londono A. Women, youth, and girls in the armed conflict. *Women and Environment International Magazine*, 2003, 58/59:25–27.

91. Amnesty International. *Sudan, Darfur, Rape as a weapon of war: sexual violence and its consequences.* London, 2004 (http://www.amnesty.org/library/index/engafr540762004, accessed 5 November 2007).

92. Pinel A, Bosire LK. Traumatic fistula: the case for reparations. *Forced Migration Review*, 2007, 27:18–19. The authors are affiliated with the United Nations Population Fund.

93. Human Rights Watch. *A question of security: Violence against Palestinian women and girls.* Issued 7 November 2006. Ramallah, occupied Palestinian territory, 2006 (http://hrw.org/reports/2006/occupied Palestinian territory1106/, accessed 4 November 2007).

94. Kakar P. *Tribal Law of Pashtunwali and Women's Legislative Authority. Afghan Legal History Project*. Islamic Legal Studies Program. Harvard Law School, 2005 (http://www.law.harvard.edu/programs/ilsp/research/alhp.php, accessed 18 December 2006).

95. Rasekh Z et al. Women's health and human rights in Afghanistan. *Journal of the American Medical Association*, 1998, 280(5):449–55.

96. Scholte WF et al. Mental health symptoms following war and repression in eastern Afghanistan. *Journal of the American Medical Association*, 2004, 292(5):585–93.

97. Freedman LP. Using human rights in maternal mortality programs: from analysis to strategy. *International Journal of Gynaecology and Obstetrics*, 2001, 75(1):51–60.

98. United Nations. UN General Assembly. *Report of the Commission of Inquiry on Lebanon, pursuant to Human Rights Council Resolution S–2/1*. Advanced unedited version. Geneva, 10 November 2006 (http://www.ohchr.org/english/bodies/hrcouncil/docs/CoI-Lebanon.pdf, accessed 5 November 2007).

99. Dugard J. *Report of the Special Rapporteur on the situation of human rights in the Palestinian territories occupied since 1967*. United Nations General Assembly. Human Rights Council, A/HRC/4/17, 29 January 2007.

100. *West Bank and the Gaza Strip: Comprehensive Food Security and Vulnerability analysis* (CFSVA). World Food Program and Food and Agriculture Organization of the United Nations, 2007.

101. *Report of the food security assessment: West Bank and the Gaza Strip*. World Food Programme and Food and Agriculture Organization of the United Nations. 2003 (http://www.fao.org//docrep/006/j1575e/j1575e00.htm, accessed 5 November 2007).

102. Siddiqi S, Masud TI, Sabri B. Contracting but not without caution: experiences with outsourcing of health services in countries of the Eastern Mediterranean Region. *Bulletin of the World Health Organization*, 2006, 84(11):867–875.

103. Mansour AA, Wanoose HL. Insulin crisis in Iraq. *The Lancet*, 2007, 369:1860.

104. Update on the health emergency in Lebanon. Regional Committee for the Eastern Mediterranean, 53rd Session. Agenda item 18(b). EM/RC53/INF.Doc.12. Cairo, WHO Regional Office for the Eastern Mediterranean, 2006 (http://www.who.int/entity/social_determinants/resources/conflcits_and_sdh_07.pdf, accessed 8 October 2008).

105. Amnesty International. *Israel/Lebanon: out of all proportion – civilians bear the brunt of the war*. Released 21/11/2006. Amnesty International UK, 2006 (http://www.amnesty.org/library/print/ENGMDE02033206, accessed 2 December 2007).

106. Human Rights Council. Report on Special Rapporteurs mission to Lebanon and Israel. UN General Assembly, Human Rights Council, Second Session, Agenda item 2A/HRC.2/7, 2 October 2006. UN, Geneva, 2006 (http://www.ohchr.org/english/bodies/hrcouncil/2session/documents.htm, accessed 20 November 2007).

107. Zurayk H, Nuwayhid I. *Can we count on a "social vaccine in war and in peace"*. Abstract of presentation at Forum 10, Global Forum for Health Research, 29 October–2 November, 2006, Cairo, Egypt, 2006.

108. Acra SA. Impact of war on the household environment and domestic activities: vital lessons from the civil war in Lebanon. *Journal of Public Health Policy*, 2006, 27:136–145.

109. Hill AG et al. Hope and despair over health in Gaza. *British Medical Journal*, 2006, 333:845–6.

110. Morris T. Just a wall? *Forced Migration Review*, 2006, 6:30 (http://www.moh.gov.ps/pdffiles/Intifada12.pdf, accessed 25 October 2007).

111. Shearer D. Territorial fragmentation of the West Bank. *Forced Migration Review*, 2006, 26:22–23. The author is Head of the UN Office for the Coordination of Humanitarian Affairs, Jerusalem.

112. Shaar AN. *Social Determinants of Health, Palestine country paper*. Cairo, WHO Regional Office for the Eastern Mediterranean, March 2006 (http://gis.emro.who.int/HealthSystemObservatory/PDF/Social%20determinants%20of%20heatlh/Palestine.pdf, accessed 8 October 2008).

113. United Nations. UN General Assembly establishes register of damage arising from construction of wall by Israel in the occupied Palestinian territory. Resolution GA/10560, 15 December 2006 (http://www.un.org/News/Press/docs//2006/ga 10560.doc.htm, accessed 17 December 2006).

114. Loewenstein J. Identify and movement control in the occupied Palestinian territory. *Forced Migration Review*, 2006, 6:24.

115. Rice X. *Smugglers push Yemen migrants into sea and leave 107 to drown*. The Guardian (UK), 2007 (http://www.guardian.co.uk/international/story/0,2015121,00.html, accessed 4 November, 2007).

116. Médecins Sans Frontières. MSF Press release: MSF is responding to cholera outbreaks in Somalia, 11 April 2007 (http://www.msf.org/msfinternational/invoke.cfm?component=pressreleaseandobjectid=E487C327-15C5-F00A-2508EBC812E4216Eandmethod=full_html, accessed 11 November 2007).

117. Ghosh N, Mohit A, Murthy RS. Mental health promotion in post-conflict countries. *Journal of the Royal Sociey for Promotion of Health*, 2004, 124(6):268–270.

118. Lowry C. Women's centres: spaces of empowerment in Darfur. *Forced Migration Review*, 2007, 27:43.

119. Anon. Listening to the women of Darfur. *Forced Migration Review*, 2006, 27:42–43. Extracts from The effects of conflict on health and well-being of women and girls in Darfur: Conversations with the community. United Nations Population Fund/UNICEF (http://unicef.org/infobycountry/files/sitan_unfpaunicef.pdf, accessed 8 October, 2008).

120. Hashim FA. Sudanese women acting to end sexual violence. *Forced Migration Review*, 2007, 27:44.

121. Sabri B et al. Towards sustainable delivery of health services in Afghanistan: options for the future. *Bulletin of the World Health Organization*, 2007, 85(9):712–719.

122. Development of a nurse-midwifery programme in Somalia. Cairo, WHO Regional Office for the Eastern Mediterranean, 2007 (unpublished).

123. Human resource development situation analysis for Afghanistan. Cairo, WHO Regional Office for the Eastern Mediterranean, 2006 (unpublished).

124. Leather A et al. Working together to rebuild health care in post-conflict Somaliland. *The Lancet*, 2006, 368(9541):119–1125.

125. Huhtanen J. Review of rebuilding Somaliland: issues and possibilities, edited by Bryden M. *African Affairs*, 2007, 106(422):165–6.

126. *Resolving conflict*. Alliance for Conflict Transformation, 2005 (http://www.conflicttransformation.org/home/resolvingconflict/tabid/55/default.aspx, accessed 13 August, 2008).